"GREAT MAN, GREAT BOOK.

The worlds of medicine and adventure are populated by heroic, inspiring figures. But Dr. Chuck Dietzen stands astride both. Few other public personalities have the incredible range of experience and the depth of commitment as this hard-working pediatrician whose influence has spread from Indianapolis to the most dangerous and threatening places on earth. As this book shows, Chuck Dietzen's story is not only inspiring, it's also breathtaking. Pint-Sized Prophets *is the amazing tale of a wise and witty man who has dedicated his life to helping the youngest and the weakest among us in some of the most obscure corners of the globe. Everything he touches turns to goodness. In fact, just reading this book will make you feel much, much better—about yourself and your own potential to serve, as well as about the brave souls who have dedicated their lives to helping others."*

—Denis Boyles, author,
Man Eaters Motel and *African Lives*
and contributing editor, *Men's Health Magazine*

"I met Dr. Chuck in 2011 and led two separate volunteer groups on Timmy Global trips to Ecuador. Dr. Chuck inspired my daughter to pursue a career in medicine. Dr. Chuck is a saint, truly one of the most dedicated, selfless, loving people I have ever met. In the Jewish faith, the highest calling is the work of Tikkun Olam, which roughly translates to 'repair of the world.' Dr. Chuck Dietzen is the embodiment of Tikkun Olam. He is one of my heroes, and I am so grateful to be a part of his life."

—Tom Rivkin, president,
Central Building & Preservation L.P.

"Dr. Chuck gave us hope for our son Jimmy walking no one else had confirmed. He reminded us to let him be a little boy, which put things in perspective. Many people have great ideas—Dr. Chuck makes them happen, i.e. the Timmy Takedown and bringing Challenger football to the local community. Proud to be his friend."

—Chooch and Marie Kennedy,
parents of former patient

"In Ecuador I watched Dr. Chuck make hundreds of kids smile while he was making them physically healthier. Most leaders spend a lifetime trying to become successful and only a short few years trying to become significant. Dr. Chuck's formula has been the complete opposite. He knew early that his calling was to care for kids and has created extraordinary ways to live this mission. That's why this is the first leadership book that I will give to my kids."

—Mike Maddock, founding partner, *Maddock Douglas, Ringleader Ventures & McGuffin Creative Group*

"There are few men who are driven to serve. Chuck is one of those few men who is not only passionate about his mission but willing to give up so much of his own life in order to fulfill his purpose, his calling. This book inspires because it is of an ordinary man, one not born of means but one very much like you and me. Yet he has silently accomplished greatness and maintained great humility in the process. A man of honor and great love, his

word is his bond. Chuck is a man among men, a hero; yet he points to the children he serves as the real heroes in life. I am so blessed that he remains my longtime friend."

—Angela Budenz, mother of former patient

"Anyone with a love for children who has experienced adversity will feel the profound messages in these writings. This book is a treasure of Dr. Chuck's personal lifetime insights and experiences. He helps us to see with clarity that the healing process is not only a function of the medical abilities of a doctor but the selfless acts of love and commitment to his patients for a deeper healing of the soul. Dr. Chuck lives by his mentor and hero, Mother Teresa's words, 'a life not lived for others is not a life.'"

—Lori and Scott Bracale, president,
Tween Brands

"Chuck and I share many of the same influences and passions. And the tone of the book is in line with a current response by Pope Francis

as well. They asked His Holiness if he thought people in the USA would follow him. The pope was humored by such a question because he knows an answer that is far better than a wrong-minded question. The pope doesn't really care if folks here in the USA follow him. He follows Jesus, and so should all good people. Not just to be Christian but to be love incarnate, period.

Dr. Chuck loves St. Francis, Mother Teresa, Pope Francis, Girzone, and his character Joshua all for the same reason. They 'get it.' God is love: the simplest of messages. That is what they follow. They follow love.

To be around any of them, to be around Chuck is to be around love."

—Anthony Levi, financial advisor,
Wells Fargo Advisors

"A very interesting read. Dr Chuck Dietzen is an inspiration to everyone that meets him!"

—Kiley Toy, Timmy volunteer
and former patient

"Dr. Chuck calls life's coincidences, 'God Winks'! Dr. Chuck is a 'God Wink,' and this book is a 'God Wink' for its readers. Thank you Dr. Chuck for your thoughts, guidance, and friendship!"

—Christopher Cleveland, founder,
ballyCANhelp.org

"Today the soul of the man my son will one day become stands as a young and watchful student of Dr. Chuck. He observes what it means to be present for those most in need, experiences what a true and purposeful life can be, and will ultimately learn that a life that humbly serves others with one's God-given talents is a life that honors God."

—Stephanie Blackwell,
Super Hero Robbie's mom

"Sometimes I find young people who are thinking of going into pediatric healthcare professions saying, 'But I care too much—I don't think I can take care of sick children.' I always think

of Dr. Dietzen and tell these young people that it is impossible to care too much—caring is what makes you the perfect person to become a pediatrician or a pediatric nurse. I know Chuck cares with his whole being. There is a wonderful quote from Henry Ward Beecher, famous Presbyterian minister in the nineteenth century: 'Children are the hands by which we take hold of heaven.'"

—Jim Lemons, emeritus professor,
Pediatrics, *Indiana University*

pint-sized —— PROPHETS

*In honor of Mom
and in memory of Dad*

pint-sized PROPHETS

INSPIRATIONAL MOMENTS
THAT TAUGHT ME
WE ARE ALL BORN TO BE HEALERS

by

DR. CHUCK DIETZEN

Advantage

Published by Advantage, Charleston, South Carolina.
Member of Advantage Media Group.

ADVANTAGE is a registered trademark and the Advantage colophon is a trademark of
Advantage Media Group, Inc.

Printed in the United States of America.

Cover photo by Dr. Joe Bergeron.

ISBN: 978-1-59932-781-5
LCCN: 2016931659

Events described in this book are based on Dr. Dietzen's memory of real-world
situations. However, certain names of patients discussed in this book, even given at all,
have been changed. Identifying details have also been changed.

This publication is designed to provide accurate and authoritative information in
regard to the subject matter covered. It is sold with the understanding that the
publisher is not engaged in rendering legal, accounting, or other professional services.
If legal advice or other expert assistance is required, the services of a competent
professional person should be sought.

Advantage Media Group is proud to be a part of the Tree Neutral® program.
Tree Neutral offsets the number of trees consumed in the production and
printing of this book by taking proactive steps such as planting trees in direct
proportion to the number of trees used to print books. To learn more about
Tree Neutral, please visit www.treeneutral.com. To learn more about
Advantage's commitment to being a responsible steward of the environment,
please visit www.advantagefamily.com/green

Advantage Media Group is a publisher of business, self-improvement, and professional
development books and online learning. We help entrepreneurs, business leaders,
and professionals share their Stories, Passion, and Knowledge to help others Learn &
Grow™. Do you have a manuscript or book idea that you would like us to consider for
publishing? Please visit advantagefamily.com or call 1.866.775.1696.

TABLE OF CONTENTS

Foreword .... *v*

Introduction *1*

PART ONE
Learning to Live a Life of Compassion *5*

CHAPTER 1
A Spiritual Quest *7*

CHAPTER 2
The Influence of Mother Teresa *29*

PART TWO
Lessons to Live By *49*

CHAPTER 3
Be Present *51*

CHAPTER 4
Be Vulnerable *77*

CHAPTER 5
Be Courageous *93*

CHAPTER 6
Be Compassionate *111*

CHAPTER 7
Be Ordinary.. *125*

CHAPTER 8
Be True... *139*

CHAPTER 9
Be Selfless... *155*

CHAPTER 10
Be Humble *169*

CHAPTER 11
Be Hopeful.. *189*

CHAPTER 12
Be Amazed...*215*

CHAPTER 13
Be an Instrument of Peace...........................*237*

CHAPTER 14
Be an Inspiration...*247*

CONCLUSION
Be Persistent...*269*

This is Life!

To be born
And to give birth
To care
And be cared for
To hold
And to be held
To feed
And be fed
To listen
And be heard
To have loved
And to have been loved
To die
And be born anew!

CD

Proceeds received from the sale of this book will support Dr. Chuck's missions both locally and globally.

Foreword

There's a reason why Dr. Chuck Dietzen calls the children he takes care of "pint-sized prophets." Each child exudes heart, courage, love, and the gift of life. So do all the stories that Dr. Chuck shares about the children who have transformed him and all the people they have touched.

The truth is, Dr. Chuck has also transformed and touched many people's lives. Yet it's a distinction he downplays, so let's just focus on the incredible bond between these children and Dr. Chuck. As an example, consider the story of a special moment between Dr. Chuck and a child named Jacob, a story that takes place on the day of an unusual wrestling match.

One of the featured wrestlers scheduled to appear in the match is a dastardly villain known as "Doctor Doom." If you look closely, you swear he bears a remarkable resemblance to Dr. Chuck. Then you realize it *is* Dr. Chuck. In fact, Dr. Chuck is a former professional wrestler and a talented athlete who also played quarterback and defensive back for college and semi-professional football teams.

As Dr. Chuck changes from his medical clothes to his wrestling costume on this day, he removes the chain holding the medal that Mother Teresa gave him when he traveled to India to help disabled children and to visit her in 1997—six months before she died. Standing inside the motherhouse, waiting to meet her, he could tell his heart rate was soaring. When Mother Teresa appeared from behind a curtain, she sat next to Dr. Chuck on a bench. Small, sick and stooped, she spent 20 minutes talking to a group of visitors, stressing the importance of giving people hope. When she finished, she paused for a photo with Dr. Chuck and gave him a card plus the miraculous medal. Later, she wrote him a letter thanking him for helping the crippled children of India. The framed letter hangs in his office, near a wall plaque that displays this quote from Mother Teresa: "I know God won't give me anything I can't handle. I just wish he didn't trust me so much."

Dr. Chuck returned from India even more inspired to help children. He had already dedicated his life to caring for children with spinal injuries, head injuries, and other disabilities. He already helped run a summer camp for children with disabilities. Now he decided to start a foundation to help children around the world. He accumulated medicines and medical equipment that were considered waste in the United States and used it to help children in countries where stringent legal liabilities weren't such a concern. More important, that foundation has evolved into Timmy Global Health with the mission to expand access to healthcare and empower students and volunteers to tackle today's most pressing global health challenges. His travels have taken him to several countries in South America, Central America, Eastern Europe, and Africa, as well as China, Cuba, Haiti, India, and Jordan. Still, Dr. Chuck downplays those efforts. Instead, he says, "The children I work with give me an incredible amount of faith."

One of those children is Jacob, the nine-year-old boy who will be the opponent of "Doctor Doom" on this day. Dr. Chuck knows how much all children need to believe in themselves and need to believe they can overcome obstacles and setbacks to do great things with their lives. So he sometimes stages elaborate wrestling matches with his young patients—scenes that often turn into classic battles where good gets the opportunity to triumph over evil, where hope fights and overcomes despair.

That scene is already taking shape in the hospital gym where the crowd showers applause on Jake the Snake, the wrestling moniker of nine-year-old Jacob. Nine months ago, Jacob nearly died. His recovery and rehabilitation now spark the cheers and the smiles of the families, friends, and staff members who have gathered for this main event, seeing in Jacob the same dreams and hopes they have for their own children, for all the children at the hospital. In the midst of that celebration, Doctor Doom—a spectacle in his black knee-high boots, black-and-red-striped shirt, and a black hood trimmed in blood red—finally rushes into the arena as the hoots and hisses of the crowd rain down on him.

Jacob's mother sits at ringside, just a few feet from the royal blue wrestling mat where Jake the Snake and Doctor Doom momentarily engage in a sneering stare-down. As she watches her son and his doctor, she remembers the night when a blood clot formed in Jacob's brain. She recalls how her son was rushed to the hospital where doctors tried to prepare her and her husband for the likelihood that their son would soon die. Even when Jacob beat the odds, the future seemed to offer little hope. He couldn't eat, swallow, talk, or move when he arrived at the children's rehabilitation facility where Dr. Chuck worked. When she saw Dr. Chuck, she asked him if Jacob's life would always be this way.

"He said no and gave me such hope," she recalls. "And that was something no one else had given me. I've never lost hope since then. Jacob can now eat, he can swallow, he can talk. But most of all, you know what Jacob can do? He can hug me. And I never thought I'd feel that again. Jacob loves Dr. Chuck and prays for him every night."

On the mat, Jake the Snake takes the upper hand in the match, leading the crowd to cheer wildly. Jacob gets Doctor Doom in a headlock. Doctor Doom counters by attacking Jacob from behind and forcing him to the mat—a dastardly move that leads the crowd to boo wildly. Escaping, Jake regains his feet and decides there's no better time to unleash his secret weapon. Reaching into the burlap sack on his hip, he throws several slimy, rubbery snakes at Doctor Doom, who is blinded for a split second—just enough for Jake the Snake to take down Doctor Doom and pin him for the victory. Cheers and laughter fill the room as Jake leaps to his feet—the champion.

Sitting in his office, after giving Jacob the championship belt, Dr. Chuck pulls at the long, black shoelaces of his knee-high wrestling boots. "When I was young, I prayed for three things," he says, "To help as many people as possible, to hurt as few as possible, and to have unshakable faith.

When I focus on the children, those things typically come my way."

He's surrounded at every turn by gifts, drawings, and keepsakes from children. A wall plaque reads, "Children are to be seen and heard and believed." A "Wrestling Champion" belt of cardboard and glitter, made by children in a Kentucky clinic, hangs on the wall.

"These kids are amazing," he says. "Look at Jacob. They were planning his funeral. They were talking about organ donation. And you saw him out there today. These children are often displayed as hopeless and helpless. But these children are magnificent spirits that happen to occupy small bodies. They radiate hope."

So does the story you are about to begin.

—John Shaughnessy

Introduction

I have the greatest job in the world. I am blessed to be the caregiver of my spiritual leaders. For the past twenty-seven years, I have served as the personal physician for many of the great gurus who have been sent here to make us better people. I am a pediatric rehabilitation doctor, and I have dedicated my career to providing for children in the United States and around the world. What I have discovered is that the children I care for are magnificent spirits that happen to occupy little bodies. In my world, those bodies are often impaired by disease or disability. Despite their obvious challenges—or maybe because of them—these children have become great teachers of wisdom for me. I

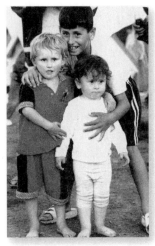

Brothers' Keeper

am truly a better person when I am in their presence. They have shown me the principles we should follow to live a more joyful life and to help heal the lives of others. In honor of all of my young heroes, and in memory of some of them, I will reveal in the following chapters the great lessons they have taught me.

—Dr. Chuck Dietzen

PART ONE

Learning to Live a Life of Compassion

CHAPTER 1

A Spiritual Quest

*"What do you want to be
when you grow up?"*

I n kindergarten, I was absolutely
sure I wanted to be a veterinarian.
And being a good Catholic boy, I didn't
want to be just *any* veterinarian; I wanted
to be the patron saint of animals, St.

Francis. I had seen statues and pictures of St. Francis standing in a field, with birds landing on him or flying around him. It wasn't uncommon for me to stand in our family's yard, holding breadcrumbs, as still as I could to see if I might draw the birds to me.

Most of my earliest memories involve taking care of animals in my neighborhood. We lived on a country road, and people brought all kinds of sick and injured animals to our house. I had a little vet clinic underneath the apple tree where I cared for them. I was not very successful, so I also had a small cemetery under the same tree. I prayed over the animals and was sure that if it were just a matter of faith, God would respond. I believed I was as faithful as I could be.

This part of my childhood wasn't just a time of developing spiritually. It was also a period of seeking affirmation. Even at such a young age, I believed that God appreciated what I was doing. There was a time when praying under that apple tree felt like something more, not exactly a vision but a type of knowing. I was convinced that I had a great spiritual mission in the world. I just couldn't completely understand it at the time. Being a sensitive, nervous kid who stuttered, I couldn't imagine myself healing or leading people.

Although God didn't always breathe life back into the sparrows, rabbits, or other animals I was praying over, I like to think he was breathing *something* into me. Years later, I realize life is not just about your beliefs. It is also about how you experience

God. I believe the best definition of God is the simplest one: God is Love.

I also believe we all need to reconnect with our innate desire to take care of people and nature. Everyone has it. When I share my story about wanting to be St. Francis and having a vet clinic and a little cemetery underneath the apple tree, people relate and respond to it. Unfortunately, as we go through this world, somehow that desire gets lost. There's so much noise and static in our world that we don't tune into our spiritual side.

Those childhood experiences were crucial in developing my spiritual mission to save lives and provide a higher quality of life for the terminally ill. My career as a doctor began underneath that apple tree, though it would take many more years for that dream to be realized.

CARING FOR THE CHILDREN

When I was seven years old, I remember standing in front of the window in our family's rec room. My mom told my siblings and me about a little boy named Mikey who didn't have a family or a home. She asked if we should invite him into our home. I thought, *He doesn't have a home? He doesn't have a mom and dad?* Growing up in my family, that was unimaginable. Mikey was two when he arrived, and he instantly had a profound impact on me. He was the first of about 150 foster children who came into our home during the next twenty years. They ranged in age from less than a day old to age sixteen.

Sometimes, when children arrived in our home, everything they owned was in a brown paper bag or even in trash bags. Years later, an organization in Indianapolis was started to give suitcases to foster children. A suitcase, at least, provides some token of dignity to the process of growing up in foster care. These kids came and went from our home. It was heartbreaking for me. Somebody once asked me, "What did you do after they came and took the children?" I would lie around for two or three days, crying. I wondered what would become of them. And I prayed they would finally be adopted by a loving family.

Of those 150 kids, we adopted two, my brother Vince and my sister Connie, both younger than me. Vince has hemophilia, a hereditary condition associated with excessive and spontaneous bleeding. If it hadn't been for the hemophilia, we probably would not have had the opportunity to adopt him, because people were fearful of that condition. In 1971, when he was born, the National Hemophilia Foundation's tagline was, "How do you tell your son it costs $21,000 each year to keep him alive?"

On the day we discussed adopting Vince, my dad sat on the couch, and we all joined him around the coffee table. Vince had been with us a few months. My dad said, "If we adopt Vince, it may take every bit of money I make to keep him alive." He was asking if we were willing to forgo everything to adopt Vince. We all raised our hands in favor of adopting Vince. Whatever we had to give up, he was worth it.

As our family cared for these foster children, my brothers, sisters, and I tried to help raise them and teach them how to act mannerly and how to treat others well. We instilled in them the idea of loving others because some of them had never known love or a loving home. The more I helped with them, the more my mom noticed I had a special way of connecting with children. When I was around twelve, she asked, "Have you ever thought about being a pediatrician? You have a gift with kids."

At the time, there were three reasons I didn't want to be a doctor. Doctors, even pediatricians, seemed too stuffy—not my kind of people. I also had no interest in hacking up a cadaver. Yet, most importantly, I couldn't imagine surviving the death of a child.

FINDING MY CALLING

Convinced that I wanted to be a veterinarian, I went to Purdue University to major in animal science. During my sophomore year, I came home just before Christmas of 1980 to find a new foster child living in our home. The little guy was a two-and-a-half-year-old who had been sent to our home because of child abuse. When I arrived at our home, I knocked on the garage door. I could see a little tyke jumping up and down yelling, "Chuckles is here! Chuckles is here! Chuckles is here!"

That was my first introduction to Matthew. He was an active, rambunctious boy. He also had a mischievous smile, piercing blue eyes, and light-colored hair with bangs cut straight across. And his giggles revealed a vibrant, life-loving spirit. When I first met him, I thought, *Man, he's pretty smart. He's got quite a vocabulary.* I also discovered he was stubborn, he didn't like to follow rules, and he was hungry for attention. We immediately started to work together. I tried to teach him some manners.

I'd say, "Hello Matthew, how are you doing?"

He'd reply, "Fine. How are you?" We'd shake hands and laugh about our mimicking good behavior. I'd snatch him up and go to the kitchen, where we'd sit and talk about our day while having a snack. Eventually, he began to call me "Daddy."

One of the things that stood out about Matthew was that he had a deep, linear scab in the middle of his forehead. I asked him, "Matthew, what happened to your head?" He said, "When mommy gets mad at me, she slams the door on my head."

That's when I began to realize I must do what I could to help children in vulnerable situations. That feeling stayed with me even when I was accepted into vet school in my third year at Purdue. As I prepared to enter vet school in the fall of 1982, I thought, "Maybe my Mom's right. Maybe my real calling is to take care of children." I did some soul searching and some of what I refer to as "P and P" (prayer and pondering). I finally called the vet school. I told the staff person at the admissions office, "I've been accepted, but I'm not sure this is what I should be doing."

I didn't want to take one of the spots my classmates could have if I didn't plan to stay in the vet school. The admission staff person said, "If you're going to turn down the acceptance, then we need it in writing." I remember thinking, *Oh, my God! That's a tough request.* I got together a letter and signed it with, "Thank you, but no thank you." I found myself sitting on the steps of Lynn Hall at Purdue with my letter declining the offer of admission. I handed them the letter, but it felt like I was handing over my life's vision.

When I withdrew from the vet school, I only needed a few credits to get my bachelor's degree. During my senior year at Purdue, I started working on a master's degree in genetics. I also drove to the admissions office of Indiana University School of Medicine in Indianapolis, where I discovered I had covered all the prerequisites to apply to medical school. I submitted my application, took the Medical College Admission Test (MCAT), and was granted an interview.

I walked into the interview room, where a professorial doctor sat across from me behind a big desk. "So how badly do you want to be a doctor?" he asked. "How many med schools did you apply to?"

"To be honest with you, sir, IU Med School's not my first choice. I can't afford to go anywhere else, so this is the only school I've applied to."

Apparently, he appreciated the honesty because I was accepted into the school. After graduating from medical school, I decided to follow my girlfriend to Alabama and train in the specialty of Physical Medicine and Rehabilitation (PM&R) at the University of Alabama at Birmingham (UAB). I found out about PM&R through reading and research and people asking me whether I'd ever thought about being a physiatrist. I'd never heard of that. The more I learned, the more I realized, "Wow! I can be a coach and a doctor, all in one. That would be a good fit for me."

Following my passion for sports, I had kept active playing semi-pro football and club rugby throughout my undergraduate and graduate years. While I trained as a doctor, I also played quarterback for the inaugural UAB football team. We had 130 players try out for the team, ten for the position of quarterback. I was chosen as the starting quarterback.

When I finished training at UAB, they offered me a position to stay on doing sports medicine and pediatric rehabilitation. But instead, I took a position at King's Daughters Medical Center and Our Lady of Bellefonte Hospital in northeastern Kentucky, as they had no board-certified physical medicine and rehabilitation doctor in that area of the state. I began work there in 1991.

While I was in Kentucky, my background in football and wrestling became known. I told people, "I know how to treat most of these injuries because I've had them." Because of the press I received, I was asked to help coach a wrestling team at a local high school. One day, I gave the wrestlers a tongue-lashing for not working hard enough in practice. After that incident, I felt I should step down from coaching.

Within a week or two, the office manager said, "Dr. Chuck, there's a Don Belt here to see you. His son, Jason, is on the wrestling team." I thought, *Oh, great. He's here to complain about what I had said.*

Don walked into my office and said, "Jason told me about your background in amateur wrestling. Would you be interested in being a pro wrestler?" He handed me his card. He was the promoter for Eastern U.S. Championship Wrestling and World of Professional Wrestling. I signed on and soon took the ring name of "Doctor

Doom." I became well known for injecting my opponents with sleeping medicine. One of my managers was a sixteen-year-old with cerebral palsy, Todd. He would get so excited that his spasticity would almost throw him out of his wheelchair. I also had another manager, Kevin, a policeman who'd been shot in the neck when he delivered a warrant. Both of my managers were wheelchair-dependent. We had a blast.

During that time, I also met a wrestling fan I'll never forget. After going to Mass one Sunday at Holy Family Church, the priest asked me if I would visit one of the parishioners in the hospital, a boy named Joey. Joey had muscular dystrophy, a disease that caused him significant difficulties breathing. The thought was he wouldn't live much longer. After being directed to his room by a nurse, I found a twelve-year-old boy with noticeable deformities, laboring to suck oxygen from a mask. He struggled to pull each breath. I sat next to the bed and started talking to him, asking him what his hobbies were. Fortunately, his mother was in the room, and she answered my questions, as her son had difficulty speaking. His mother said he loved sports. When I asked which one was his favorite, she said he especially loved pro wrestling. She said he was disappointed because he wouldn't be able to go to the pro wrestling show in town that weekend.

I leaned toward Joey and said, "I know you are not going to believe this, but do you know who I am?" He feebly shook his head. I said, "I am Doctor Doom." He appeared not to believe me, but his mother exclaimed that she had read a newspaper article about me being a pro wrestler.

That weekend, I participated in the wrestling show. As I entered the locker room, I told the sixteen wrestlers about Joey. They all seemed moved by his story. I also told them that, following the show, I would be happy to lead them to the hospital if they wanted to visit Joey. After the show, I waited in the parking lot. No other wrestlers came for a long time. Finally, a few showed. Thinking they would meet me there, I drove to the hospital. Yet when I entered Joey's room, there were no other wrestlers. After waiting a long time, I went into the hall and asked the nurses if they had seen any of the pro wrestlers. They said, "No, none of them has arrived." I was disappointed because I was certain they were going to show up. I went back in and sat with Joey, knowing how much it would have meant to him if the wrestlers had come. Then there came a knock on the door.

Three wrestlers entered Joey's room, soon followed by several more. Before long, twelve of the sixteen wrestlers had come to see Joey, filling up the room. They were late because they had been busy collecting wrestling memorabilia for him. Some had even stopped at the gift shop to buy him balloons. Joey couldn't believe it. He loved every minute of it.

One week later, I had to leave the city to do consulting work in another state. Joey was still in the hospital. As I sat on the plane, I asked God to send an angel to Joey, to make him feel comfortable, especially if the time came for him to die. And, if God didn't mind, I asked him to let me know he had answered my prayer. When I returned from my trip, there was a note on my office desk saying that Joey had passed away. Although it was two in the morning, I called his mother. She told me that Joey had passed peacefully.

After Mass the following day, I talked to the priest who had first asked me to visit Joey. I told him I had a long, beautiful conversation with Joey's mother. The priest said, "It was interesting what Joey's father had to say, wasn't it?" I said, "I didn't get to talk to Joey's father. What did he say?" The priest told me that Joey's father had spent the last twenty-four hours at Joey's bedside. Joey kept asking his father who the person standing in the corner was while his father kept saying no one else was in the room.

God had sent Joey an angel. And he let me know my prayer was answered.

CHAPTER 2

The Influence of Mother Teresa

The connection between faith and healthcare in my life became even more intense after that experience with Joey. A short time later, I was called to Indianapolis to work with the kids at Lifelines Children's Hospital. The administration had heard me speak at a conference.

I discussed the importance of giving kids with disabilities opportunities to participate in activities that interested them, regardless of the perceived limitations caused by their disabilities.

That experience in Indianapolis turned into a full-time job caring for the children. While I was at Lifelines Children's Rehabilitation Hospital, it was purchased by St. Vincent's Hospital and became the St. Vincent Pediatric Rehabilitation Center.

There was a great need for a pediatric hospice program. I thought our facility was a good fit because our staff knew how to do home care for medically fragile children, we knew how to support their families, and we knew the importance of spiritual care. We took a philosophical approach to support families with children who were going to die. We didn't just provide medical care. We provided spiritual care.

Our hospital was a sacred place. Children came there to learn to live, or they came there to die. To this day, whenever I talk about that place to any of the nurses, doctors, therapists, maintenance staff, or cooks that were there, we all tear up. It was a haven for children with disabilities and serious chronic diseases. It was also a haven for their families and for us. We looked forward to the weekends being over so we could be back together at the hospital. We were a family.

While I was working there, I started taking care of my heroes. Michael was one of them. He was an eight-year-old boy who had cancer. For more than a year, he had been in the children's hospital receiving multiple treatments to try to stop the growth of the disease. When he was finally transferred to our facility, he was looking forward to undergoing rehabilitation because it would allow him to return home to be with his friends and family. They had been limited in their visits because of his inability to fight infection. When Michael was admitted, he and I immediately hit it off. He had a great cantankerous spirit. He also obviously enjoyed his ability to call the shots from his hospital bed.

The weekend after he was admitted, I was driving around Indianapolis on my motorcycle. I had on tennis shoes, blue jeans, a T-shirt, and my helmet. When I was urgently paged to the hospital, I drove there, jumped off the motorcycle, and ran into the building. Fortunately, I had a baseball cap to cover my helmet hair. After stabilizing the little girl I was paged to see, I decided to stop to say hello to Michael.

He looked at me and said, "What are you wearing?!"

I said, "What? I am wearing a T-shirt, blue jeans, and a ball cap."

He said, "You're a doctor! You are supposed to be dressed up!"

I said, "Hey, buddy, this isn't the Mayo Clinic."

He replied, "I would like to talk to your boss."

Unknown to Michael, I was the medical director. But I left the room, stepped into the hallway, put on a lab coat and took off my hat, adjusted my hair, stepped back into the room, looked at Michael, and said, "Hello, Mr. Smith, I understand you are having a problem with one of our doctors." He laughed, and then we discussed how he thought I should dress more professionally the next time I visited him.

Tuesday seemed to be the best time to dress up for Michael, as I had a shorter time in the clinic on that day. When I got up Tuesday morning and began putting on my suit, it occurred to me that Michael would get the biggest kick out of me wearing a tuxedo. I knew this would lead to some uncomfortable encounters in the afternoon because I had to do a consultation at another children's hospital. But I decided I was only trying to impress Michael that day. So I put on my tuxedo and my black patent leather shoes and went to work.

Michael laughed when he saw me. And I laughed with him. But I was also hoping to share a lesson with him. I often tell people that children need to know the rules we have can be bent—and even broken—especially if it will benefit them. And I wanted him and each of the other children to know they were that important.

That goal inspired me in 1997 to start Timmy Global Health, a foundation to help children around the world. The organization is a living legacy to my hospice patients. It was originally called the Timmy Foundation. Some people wanted me to call it the Dietzen Foundation, but I didn't want to put my name or the family name on it. I wanted a foundation that helped and encouraged children, and I wanted its name to reflect that purpose. At first, I looked at the names of all the hospice patients for whom I provided care. Could I take the first letter off of each name? Could I make up a name that way? Ultimately, I decided I would call it Timmy Foundation, after my brother who died as a newborn. I approached my parents and asked, "What do you think? Are you okay with this?" My parents gave me their blessing.

We have twenty employees now, yet we maintain an overhead of less than 7 percent. Our primary concerns are recruitment and retention of people who genuinely care about making the world a better place and who are not motivated by money. We give people a fair salary, but they need to be motivated by compassion. We also have more than a thousand volunteers helping the underserved in countries around the world and several thousand more working within this country.

I'm often asked, "Did you ever think that Timmy would get this big?" I answer, "Yes, actually I did. I was certain it would." I used to tell our first executive director, when we discussed what we're doing and where Timmy was going, "I think this is destined to become huge. This is something the world needs."

A BLESSING FROM MOTHER TERESA

In 1996, I was still the medical director of the pediatric rehab center, and I was also on the trauma team at Riley Children's Hospital in Indianapolis. I did medical rounds there once a week and worked with all the residents from the IU Physical Medicine and Rehabilitation program. They trained with me to do their pediatric rehabilitation rotations.

Dr. Joe Bergeron was one of those doctors who trained with me. Joe was a former pastor of a nondenominational church in California. I thought, *I hope he's not a teetotaler.* I had promised some people we would have a "happy hour" the following week. Joe came and had a drink, and we hit it off. While we were talking, he asked, "Do you know anybody who would help me set up medical missions to India?" I simply replied, "Sure. I will."

We went to India for the first time in January 1997. I worked at a rehabilitation camp. The kids were so spastic from cerebral palsy and spinal cord or brain injuries that the mothers walked them in on the tops of their own feet. They also rolled them into the clinic in wheelbarrows because they didn't have wheelchairs. I saw 150 kids on that trip and tried to identify which of the patients were good candidates for surgical intervention.

During that first visit, we were close to where Mother Teresa and her sisters cared for people.

I tried to meet with her, but I was told she was sick at the time with back pain. I thought, *Back pain is one of the things we specialize in. I'd be glad to help, but I don't want to impose.*

I said to one of the sisters, "Look, she doesn't even need to know I'm here. I can just crawl in there and kiss her hands." Ever since I had read about Mother Teresa and all the people she had touched, I wondered, *How many people have those hands lifted out of the gutter? How many people has she bathed and nursed back to health with those hands?*

While I didn't get to meet her on that trip, I did what I thought was the next best thing. I ran to the Sisters of Saint Paul Bookstore, which sold rosaries. I bought

176 rosaries, all the rosaries they had. I asked one of the Missionaries of Charity sisters, "Could you please take these to Mother Teresa and ask her to bless them for me? I would be very thankful." She did. Mother Teresa blessed the rosaries and wrote on a little card, "God bless you, Dr. Chuck Dietzen." I wanted to bring back as many rosaries as I could for my family and all my patients.

About six weeks later, I received a phone call, insisting that I return to India as soon as possible to meet Mother Teresa. I headed back as quickly as I could.

MEETING MOTHER TERESA

When I returned to India in March 1997, I met Mother Teresa in an area of the Mother House on Circular Road in Calcutta. It was a hot, humid day. I stood in a little entryway, with a blue-and-white checkered cloth hanging over the doorway. It looked like a tablecloth. Eventually, a nun stepped from behind the cloth and said, "Take a seat. Mother will be here shortly."

My heart raced, 180 to 190 beats per minute. I hadn't had that feeling since the night before I ran with the bulls in Pamplona, Spain, in 1995. I couldn't sleep that night, because I was certain I would get killed the next day. I had put running with the bulls on my "bucket list" when I was a teenager so I had to do it. My increased heart rate could also have been caused by my anxiety over a possible pending career change. One of the nuns told me that Mother may ask me to become a priest since I wasn't married. I decided, prior to meeting Mother Teresa, that that would be my omen. If she had requested I join the priesthood, I decided I would go to the seminary. I sat down, thank God, because it would have been bad form to pass out in front of Mother Teresa. I sat on this little bench, no more than three feet long. I didn't expect a red carpet and trumpets, but I thought there would be some formality to meeting her. Instead, she just pulled the tablecloth aside and stepped out. The only place for her to sit was right next to me.

I had a micro-cassette recorder and her book. I wanted to ask her to sign the book, but I didn't want to

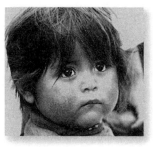

Dirty, Snot-nosed, and Beautiful

impose. I wanted to turn on the recorder, catch her voice, and capture everything she said. I wish I had. At the time, it just didn't seem appropriate. She talked with us about HIV infection and AIDS. Mostly, she stressed the importance of giving hope and comfort to patients.

"No matter what you're confronted with, never abandon your patients," Mother Teresa said. "Stay there. Be their hope. Just don't abandon them. Let them know someone cares. Despite possible harm to yourself, remain there as a symbol of hope for them."

Mother Teresa always believed that God put her in the right places to help. I sometimes think of the unusual places God has put me. In 1997, I played quarterback for Team USA, a football squad made up of semi-pro and college players who toured the world playing other national teams and semi-pro teams. We played in Hawaii in the spring of that year. One of the people from that football team I'll never forget was the offensive coordinator. It's not uncommon for football coaches to be described as aggressive and even angry at times, but this coach was especially irate, often screaming in practice.

After practice one day, we returned to our hotel at the same time. He and I had adjacent rooms. When we were keying into our rooms, the coach surprised me when he said, "I heard that you worked with Mother Teresa." I told him of the blessing I had received in March of that year when working in India. I told him I had met with Mother Teresa, and she had sent me a letter after I returned to the United States. He proceeded to tell me he had a fourteen-year-old son who had cerebral palsy. His son would never play football. As we talked, he made it clear how angry he was with God. It didn't even seem to comfort him when he told me his son could play the piano well.

Nothing dramatic happened that day to change his anger. I, and the team, performed poorly that weekend. Still, after returning home, I forwarded some books to the coach—and a medal given to me by Mother Teresa. From later correspondence with him, I believe he found some peace—with God, his son's situation, and most importantly, himself. It became clear to me that this coach was the reason I was in Honolulu. It had nothing to do with playing football, but the game brought us together.

I believe we're here to reach out in compassion to one another, to help one another.

I've learned that approach from being with Mother Teresa. Most of all, I've learned it from the children I call "my gurus." Now, I want to share their wisdom with you.

PART TWO

Lessons to Live By

CHAPTER 3

Be Present

I'm the caregiver of my spiritual leaders. These children have helped me discover what is truly important to me. They have shaped how I live my life. They have led me to consider deeply this question, "What principles do I have to follow if I want to make a difference?"

I now understand that the first principle is, "Be present." To be present means being there with others physically, mentally, and spiritually—without distraction or interruption. To be a healer for these children demands my full attention while I am in their presence.

When I teach at the medical center, I walk along the hallways and often see doctors, nurses, and therapists -- all with their faces hidden behind computers. We're reimbursed for documenting that we gave quality care. Whether we did or not is immaterial when you consider today's medicolegal issues. As I train future doctors, I tell them, "You must take the risk of stepping close enough to the fire to be burned." That means forcing yourself to come close to the bedside. These days, we have plenty of technology, medicines, procedures, and surgical techniques that are at our disposal. They allow us to distance ourselves from the patients. Yet, the most important lessons we must learn are at the bedside. We must be caring and compassionate enough to not walk away from that bedside. Walking away is easy to do, but we need to stay.

Years ago, I dropped my membership with the American Medical Association (AMA). One of the editorial board members of the *Journal of the American Medical Association* (JAMA) wrote an editorial suggesting that everyone training to become a doctor should take an acting class so he/she could appear to be a compassionate, caring individual despite his/her busy schedule. My reaction was, "You don't think a patient will see through that? You don't think when people are in need, they will realize whether or not you are genuine and sincerely interested in their well-being?" I never joined the AMA again.

In today's world, much of our communication is done with text and e-mail, but in any communication course you take in college you learn that 90 percent of communication is nonverbal. If you're going to support or help heal someone, you have to be present in each moment with the patient. I learned that with my first patient.

When I began my clinical rotations as a third-year medical student in 1985, the first child ever assigned to me was Abby. She was a three-year-old girl who had been diagnosed with

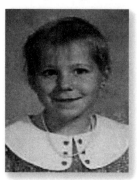

Abby, my first patient, was given less than a 10 percent chance of survival.

leukemia and lymphoma. Her arms and legs were no bigger around than a silver dollar, but her belly was large because cancer cells filled her liver and spleen. Her prognosis was poor. She was given less than a 10 percent chance of survival.

The greatest fear I had about becoming a doctor—that a child under my care would die—confronted me with my very first patient.

During that time, I noticed that doctors and nurses tended to avoid patients who were expected to die. Yet, I felt the opposite with Abby. I found myself pulled toward this little girl who often struggled with fevers and the side effects of the chemotherapy she received. I sat with her in the evenings, reading books to her and telling her stories. Sometimes, I would run to a nearby McDonald's to get her a hamburger and fries because she wouldn't eat most of the food that was delivered at her bedside from the hospital kitchen.

The staff doctor and resident physicians would call the nurses in the evenings and instruct them to tell me to leave the hospital when I came to see Abby. They feared that when Abby did die, it would break my heart. They worried I might not complete my training. I remember having a different feeling: Even if Abby didn't survive, her spirit would. I also did not feel I needed to be protected from death. I thought it was more important that as she approached death, I should be there for her and her family. I also imagined being in Abby's position. I believed it would be scary if people suddenly stopped coming to visit and spent less time with me.

So I kept visiting Abby. And here's the best part of the story—she beat the odds. Abby is now thirty-three. She has four children. She lived, and she brought life into the world. We can measure most of the effects of treatment with our medications and procedures, but how will we ever measure the positive impact of our mere presence on a person's recovery?

Abby and I have remained friends all

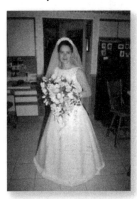

these years. To this day, I still carry her picture in my wallet. I show it to medical students and other healthcare professionals who are in training.

Abby on her wedding day

I tell them that being present for patients is the most

important part of what we do. This is why we should be invested. This is why we should feel called to do the work we are doing. Ultimately they will find, as I did, that the patient and the doctor heal each other.

We can't always cure these children, but we can heal them; we can instill in them that they are of great value and have great gifts to share. They give us hope, and a sense of what humanity is supposed to be. They draw out the love within us.

WHEN JOY SHINES THROUGH THE SUFFERING

When we experience a connection with other people, we're learning to be what we're meant to be; we're learning to be human. We should allow ourselves to have more intimacy with others, to fully feel pain and loss. We should also open ourselves to the joy in our lives, including the joy that sometimes shines through in the midst of suffering. Happiness is the weather; joy is the climate. There will not be growth without sunshine and rain. That's what these children have taught me.

It's painful sometimes to do this work, but even during the lowest points, we get to celebrate life. To be with these families, even after the loss of a child, is remarkable. The experience forever shapes how we approach the world and how forgiving we become. I had a patient named Brandon. He died before he was a year old. He had a disease, which

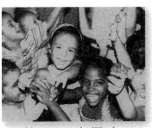

Happiness is the Weather; Joy is the Climate

caused him to have seizures that led to his death. At his memorial service, I asked the people there to look at Brandon's casket. Then I said, "When we look down at a short casket, we should remind ourselves how short a period of time we have here. We need to look around the church and see how full it is. Brandon had touched that many of us in such a short time. So rather than ask ourselves, 'Why does this happen to children?', the question should be, 'If you subtract his age from ours, have we touched as many people as he did with all the additional years we were granted?'"

A short while after Brandon's funeral, his mother wrote me a letter. In part of it, she noted, "Brandon only lived for eleven months and twelve days, but he taught me more about love and life during that time than I had learned in a lifetime. I learned to love God more and more as the days went on. I realized that Brandon was God's before he was mine. I know I never have to worry about Brandon because I know he is safe in the arms of Jesus." She also told me about a local couple in her community who had a newborn baby that started having seizures and how the child was rushed in an air ambulance to a hospital. She and her husband drove ninety minutes to be with the parents of the newborn, to offer them their support.

When we step into such circumstances, feel for these people, and take the risk to say to God, "Take some suffering away from this child and give it to

> *Take some suffering away from this child and give it to me.*

me," it leads to phenomenal spiritual growth that we can't get in any other way.

IN SEARCH OF SPIRITUAL WEALTH

I remember reading a quote when I was a kid, "You don't remember days, you remember moments." The only way that we hold onto those moments are as snapshots in our minds that bring back joy and sometimes sorrow. In 1993, I began doing a lot of work in Haiti. I went there two or three times a year for several years until I became involved in work in other countries. After my first trip to Haiti, someone asked, "Chuck, what was the most remarkable experience down there? What do you remember most?" They thought I would mention a particular case.

Even though I saw human suffering as I had never experienced it previously, I told them, "I learned the inverse relationship between material wealth and spiritual wealth. So much of what's going on in our culture is static."

> *I learned the inverse relationship between material wealth and spiritual wealth.*

We are not tuning into the spiritual realm of our lives. We are not tuning into each other, because we have so many distractions: phones, radios, TVs, computers. Most homes or businesses have all kinds of media firing away. It's easy to allow yourself to be distracted from what's important—namely, other people.

A young woman that I knew, Sierra, once wrote a short essay titled, "The Last Stitch."

The Last Stitch
By Sierra VanderKelen

"I'll hold here, and you just snip right in-between," Dr. Chuck calmly explained to me. Easier said than done. My hand was shaking uncontrollably. I knew it was basically impossible for me to mess up taking out a stitch, but my hand was refusing to behave. I took a few deep breaths and looked at Dr. Chuck, who was grinning and nodding in a manner as to say, "You've got this." I decided to just go for it.

Dr. Chuck pulled on the stitch giving me a nice area to cut, but right as the tips of my scissors were about to touch the stitch, I had to pull back. The little boy's forehead had begun dripping blood. I knew he was bleeding because I was taking too long. "It's just a scab, it's supposed to bleed," Dr. Chuck assured me. But it was too late to console me, my eyes were already filling up with water and I was ready to stop. I glanced down at the four-year-old Ecuadorian boy in his Buzz Lightyear tee shirt *Why is Dr. Chuck letting me do this? I thought, I'm not a doctor; I can't do this.* I attempted to ask him, but the words wouldn't come out of my mouth.

I wanted to do this. I wanted to know that I helped this little boy. I wanted to make his forehead stop bleeding. I craved the possibility of a patient genuinely thanking me for helping, rather than thanking me for just observing. I didn't want to disappoint Dr. Chuck, the person who not only truly believed I could do this, but also felt I could follow in his footsteps someday; the person who felt like a part of my family only after a few days.

It dawned on me: today was my last day with Dr. Chuck.

I wasn't ready for this to be my last day. My mind went into a whirlwind of thought about having to go back to America and having to put my dreams, which had finally reached their full potential, on hold once again. I wished to stay beside Dr. Chuck—the founder of the organization that I had traveled with to Ecuador. I wanted to hear more of his stories about the countless people he's helped in a myriad of countries. Ever since he became a doctor he has given up over 8 weeks each year to helping people in impoverished countries. He even worked alongside Mother Teresa on and off for two years. He has sacrificed so much of his time helping others that he has never been married or had children. Instead, his family and his children are the people he works with and inspires on a daily basis. While he isn't traveling helping people in other countries, he strives towards helping children in his community by being a pediatric physical medicine and rehabilitation specialist. He is the first truly selfless person I have ever met, and was about to disappear from my life for a whole year. He was the first person to sincerely assure me I was capable of becoming a doctor and made me believe it whole-heartedly. I wasn't ready to return to the reality that working in medical clinics, and being mentored by Dr. Chuck, was not my life.

I knew the first step to keeping these experiences a part of my life later on, was finishing the task at hand. So, I looked directly at the little boy's forehead, steadied my hand, and, in a second, the stitch was out. I had done it. I had taken out the stitch. I could feel the corners of my lips pinching my cheeks. I was ecstatic. Dr. Chuck smiled at me in congratulations as I shook the little boy's hand. He had been the 120th patient of the day; we were done.

In this essay, she talked about me, my experience working with Mother Teresa, and how I view the whole world as my family. The greatest satisfaction I get comes from stepping back and spending time with one of the young people I'm mentoring or healing. It's an awesome sensation to see young people—disabled or not—suddenly realize just how valuable they are.

I had a patient named David. When he was ten, he was ready to begin another season in the Challenger Little League, a program that allows children ages six to eighteen to play baseball regardless of their disability. During our first day of practice, all the rookies were sitting in their wheelchairs or standing with their walkers, braces, and crutches as we introduced the coaches and talked about the league. David was there, too. He had been playing in the league for five years. After all the coaches were introduced, I told the players, "Any of you who are rookies who have questions might want to talk to David here. He is the seasoned veteran." With that, we broke up to practice hitting and throwing.

Later, I saw David standing in the outfield talking to some of the rookies as they were throwing the ball back and forth. I went out and asked David how things were going.

He said, "Pretty good I guess, but my feet are hurting."

I said, "Well, why don't you sit down?"

He said, "I can't. I'm the seasoned veteran."

I suggested that we walk to the backstop and he could sit on the bleachers. From there, he could coach the batting and no one would have to know his feet hurt. So we began walking to the infield. As we got between first and second base, David looked up at me and said, "Could I get 'Seasoned Veteran' put on my shirt?"

I tell some of my patients, "I don't know how to explain this to you, but to God you are worth everything he's ever created. Your self-worth needs to be based on that truth." When you can help make that rev- 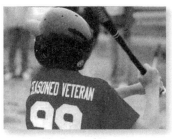 elation come

The Seasoned Veteran

true for patients, so they suddenly see themselves as powerful souls with a meaning, mission, and worth—I don't know what could be more rewarding.

> *To God you are worth*
> *everything he's ever created.*

HOW I STAY PRESENT

My inspiration to stay present is Mother Teresa. As I mentioned earlier, when I was

71

a kid, it was Saint Francis. When I began to read about Mother Teresa, I thought, *That's it! That's how you're supposed to live life.* It's not easy. There are times when I'm hustling, when I'm working eighteen-hour days or longer, and I think, *I just need to get some rest. I need to go home. I need some time to myself.* Inevitably, there is always a patient who crosses my path, stops me from hustling down the hallway, and helps renew my belief that this work is far more important than my own comfort.

I've gone through long periods when I spent a lot of time alone but was not, necessarily, lonely. I contemplate. Mother Teresa divided the Missionaries of Charity into the active branch and the contemplative branch, but she also acknowledged that the active branch is contemplative because those missionaries think and pray about what they are doing. They pray as they do their work.

What we are doing here, on this planet, is spiritual. We talk about dividing the secular and the sacred, but I don't see a difference. They should be woven together. Be aware and remind yourself that inconveniences and distractions can lead to great moments and memories.

That's how I met Jack late one night. I was about to head home after a long day at the hospital. The nurse informed me that my new patient who had suffered a stroke had been admitted. Stepping into the room, I found an older gentleman lying

> *Inconveniences and distractions can lead to great moments.*

in the bed, his features silhouetted by the overhead light. He had white hair, and he was brown-skinned with great American Indian features. I took one look at him and thought, *What a distinguished-looking man.* He was very depressed.

We exchanged a few words, and I found out he played football at Carlisle College, where one of the greatest athletes of the twentieth century, Jim Thorpe, played. I pulled up a chair and plopped myself down next to him. I said, "Jack, I was supposed to have played ball with you. I'm living at the wrong time. Tell me all about it."

We started talking, and during the conversation he told me how he had worked for a metal fabricating company.

"Well, Doc, you wouldn't know about this," he said. "I used to run the sheers."

"Jack, I used to clean the sheers at Moon Fabricating in Kokomo."

We looked at each other, smiled, and held up our hands. We laughed as we revealed we both still had all of our fingers. Lots of people lost parts of their hands in those machines. We were immediate friends. Suddenly, I wasn't as tired. It was well worth spending two more hours in the hospital, being present for Jack and myself. We stayed friends until his death.

His daughter once came to me and said, "You don't know how important it was to my dad, how you guys connected that first night."

It was important to me, too.

CHAPTER 4

Be Vulnerable

SACRED SUSCEPTIBILITY

I love my patients. They make me a better person. When I was younger, I often prayed that God would make me weak enough to feel the pain and strong enough to make a difference. I didn't realize I was actually praying for vulnerability. But somehow I realized that if I did not connect at an intimate level with those I was asked to heal, I would not be motivated to bring everything necessary to my patients. I eventually began to pray that God would just use me as a vector, a conduit, of healing for my patients. It's an incredible feeling when that sensation is realized. It is now obvious to me that healing is a mutual experience, as both lives are forever changed after such an encounter.

> *I often prayed that God would make me weak enough to feel the pain and strong enough to make a difference.*

I have recently experienced this vulnerability at a very personal level. My mom has been diagnosed with dementia. My siblings and I had been taking turns caring for her in the evenings and overnight. It was a clear revelation of life going full circle. As I helped my mother into bed one night, I realized how pleased I was that I was there to cover her legs, tuck the blanket under her chin, and give her a goodnight kiss. That moment illuminated the desire that I had that healthcare would be more like this throughout my career. I am certain that all of us healthcare providers would prefer more vulnerable, healing moments like that than working on documents.

LESSONS FROM LOSS

My work in pediatric hospice taught me that grief is additive. As each child passed on, I recognized that I was grieving not only for that child but all those that had gone before. I have to live with the hope and expectation that I will see them again. I remember telling one mother that I envisioned my brother Timmy was on the other side waiting to receive her son. The children have taught me: Eternity is a moment; eternity is a millennium.

On one occasion, I was asked to see a fifteen-year old boy with muscular dystrophy, as the pulmonologist felt he was coming to the end of life. As I entered the darkened hospital room, Andy and his mother sat quietly, not connecting with me or each other. Andy had very poor eye contact and appeared to be clinically depressed. I asked him what he liked to do, and I received no response. Finally I said, "What's something you would like to do that would scare the hell out of your mom?"

He responded that he had heard they could send your remains into space after death. I told him I was certain that he was not going any time soon so we needed to focus on how he could enjoy life.

I contacted a friend of mine who is a geologist. He supplied me with some meteorites. I gave those to Andy and told him that since he wasn't going to space any time soon, I brought space to him. Eventually, he became more interactive and told me that he always thought it would be cool to have a monkey run all over his body, as he still had normal sensation but little to no movement. We arranged for him to meet Chili, a kinkajou, at a pet shop. Chili is a

> *Eternity is a moment; eternity is a millennium.*

nocturnal animal and prefers dark spaces, so she ran into his shirt, ran all over him, eventually popping her head out of his shirt collar. She then used her long tongue to lick into his ears. Andy laughed and giggled throughout the whole experience.

HEART-TUGGING HEROES

Jimmy was two and a half years old when I met him. He has cerebral palsy, but more importantly, he has two remarkable parents who love him dearly. I don't believe I've ever seen three people enjoy each other's company more than they do. In his first clinic visit, his mother asked if he would ever be able to walk. I said, "Of course he will!" Immediately the tears streamed from his mother's eyes. As I grabbed for the

Kleenexes, I looked at Jimmy's father, a big, burly guy that looked rough around the edges. He whispered, "She's the sensitive type," as the tears began to form in his eyes. Ultimately, Jimmy's mother wrote a book, *My Perfect Son Has Cerebral Palsy*. It's the only book I had on my required reading list for the doctors I train.

Donald was a teenager who died from complications of his longstanding disease. He had very limited movement due to cerebral palsy, but he always had a ready smile and radiant eyes. He thoroughly enjoyed performing in our pro wrestling events. His mother, Donna, called me as he was coming closer to passing over. She informed me that he had seen most everybody she thought he would want to see before leaving the earth. Donna thought I was who he was waiting to see before his soul's departure. I went to their home, cupped his head, leaned forward, and whispered to him that it was okay with all of us if he wanted to move on. I told him we would come to see him in the future. He died later that night.

> It was okay with all of us if he wanted to move on.

VIGILANT FOR KIDS

In my practice, I often have victims of child abuse on my unit or in my clinic. I've seen appalling disability and death from abuse. When children are not nurtured in a safe environment, they too often experience trauma such as gunshot wounds, burns, traumatic brain injuries, and shaken infant syndrome. It frustrates me that some

people who bring children into this world
don't feel obligated to protect and care for
them. Parents and
other adults should
be helping these kids
grow and develop
instead of harming
and neglecting them.
I'm reminded of
Mikey, the first of the
foster children who

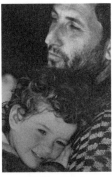

Vigilant Father

came to our home when I was a kid. It's
at the core of my being to ensure that care
for children be provided properly so they
can become the people they're meant to be,
protected from abuse and neglect.

I had a patient named Billy. He came to
one of our camps. He was ten at the time
and diagnosed with quadriplegia and was
dependent on a ventilator for breathing.

His story was especially disturbing when I discovered that his spinal cord injury occurred from child abuse by his parents. Fortunately, he was adopted by a very loving family and was enjoying a great quality of life despite his disability. He drove around in a sip-n-puff wheelchair. He also thrived in all of the camp activities, including archery, tree-climbing, and fishing with a sip-n-puff fishing pole. He particularly enjoyed the talent show. On the last night of camp, as Billy got into bed, I told him I was glad to have met him because he was such a neat kid.

He replied, "I know."

So I asked him, "Someone has told you that before?"

"I just heard it," he said.

I said, "Oh, you've heard it?"

"Yeah."

"From whom?"

"From me."

It pleased me to hear him voice his self-esteem despite suffering disability at the hands of his own parents.

SACRED VOW

It is true: Courage is fear that prays. Our team of four was transporting needed supplies to the Kosovar refugees across the Adriatic Sea in 1999. We could hear the NATO bombers overhead as we brought the supplies to the cargo ship on the southeastern coast of Italy. The truck driver asked where we were going. We responded, "Durres, Albania." With that, he muttered a response. The interpreter did not translate his comment for us. My travel companion asked what he said. The interpreter retorted, "Nothing."

She repeated, "What did he say?"

"He said nothing."

Annoyed, my companion said, "I want to know what he said."

At that, the interpreter said, "He said 'They will cut your throats for what you have.'"

With that, we loaded the supplies onto the ship. And I began a long night of prayer, as I didn't know if the other shore would be D-Day or Coney Island. Thankfully we were warmly received and assisted in our work. Obviously we were being informed by the prejudice of the Italian truck driver.

We all need to quit being so self-centered. We need to be what we say we are. We always talk about our concerns for the future of the world and how we want a better world for our children. It's easy to say, but when I look at what politicians are doing and the policies they create, they seem more concerned about the next election than what we are preserving for these kids. We in the nonprofit world need to make sure we are not experiencing mission drift. Mission drift is typically described as not remaining focused on the organization's original mission. In fact, I believe mission drift is the insidious movement of an organization's efforts to meeting their own needs rather than the needs of those they are serving. We must reflect daily on whether we are helping or exploiting those who depend on us. The line between helping and exploiting is, at times, very thin.

In the early days of Timmy Global Health, my parents asked why I had such an affinity for Quito, Ecuador. I told them the sense of community there reminded me of the relationships we enjoyed as children in our family. Family, church, and community were interdependent. All three need to be healthy institutions for the world to be a more hopeful place. We seem to have lost those foundations. Padre Carollo, the priest who founded Tierra Nueva in Ecuador, and his fellow workers assured the preservation of these three institutions and, thus, the focus of their mission.

Mission drift is the insidious movement of an organization's efforts to meeting their own needs rather than the needs of those they are serving.

CHAPTER 5

Be Courageous

I have been practicing in the specialty of pediatric physical medicine and rehabilitation for more than twenty years. I have patients with cerebral palsy and other disabilities who travel the world with me. They help heal children in other countries. Some of these children wouldn't be alive without our medical technology. Years ago,

I said, "We weren't all born to be doctors and nurses, but we were all born to be healers." I didn't think it was profound at the time, but they put it on the Timmy Global Health literature. People seemed moved by that statement.

We weren't all born to be doctors and nurses, but we were all born to be healers.

I encourage the youth I take care of to live fully. "Don't sit at home and let the government send you a disability check," I tell them. "The world will be a better place if you're out in it. Go out there and make your mark." They should have fulfilling lives. They need to make a contribution.

To do otherwise would be to allow their circumstances to take away their dignity.

It takes a lot of courage to step out there, to get in the game. It also takes encouragement.

We have to encourage the children by helping to create the stage upon which they will present their abilities. The focus should be on their abilities—not their disabilities.

I've often walked into exam rooms to meet with young men and women and their parents. They're in high school. We talk about the wheelchair. Is that working okay? How about medications? Are they okay? Where are they going to go to college? The young adults light up, almost as though they haven't thought about college at all. Mom and Dad sure haven't thought about it. They almost fall off their chairs when I introduce the subject. The question helps them move one step closer to the next journey in their lives.

I consider life to be an amazing journey. I've always wondered why I got to do all of these crazy, wonderful things that make no sense for a doctor to be doing. Professional wrestling, football, the people I've met, places I've traveled. Why did any of that make sense? It made sense because I was opening doors for my patients' futures.

When I'm kneeling next to a little girl in a wheelchair, and she looks at me and asks, "Dr. Chuck, did you live your dreams?"

I say, "Yes!"

Then, I ask, "What are yours?"

When she tells me, my mind begins turning. *Who do I know that can make sure she lives her dreams, too?*

During a medical outreach mission in Kenya, I had the opportunity to float above the Masai Mara Plains in a hot air balloon. As we looked at the wildlife below, I told several people on the balloon ride about a girl I knew, Erin. Erin was one of our campers at the first annual CHAMP Camp. CHAMP is an acronym for "Children Have A lot of Motivation and Potential." The camp was created for children who are ventilator dependent because of disease or injury or children who need technological support to survive. Our goal was to help them have as normal, no … supranormal, a childhood experience as possible.

Erin was very short in stature. She had very short limbs, a small trunk, and some facial deformities. Yet Erin also had one of the most beautiful and inspiring spirits I have encountered. She often grew tired during the course of a day, but she didn't want to miss any of the camp activities. She would always request that she could take a nap between activities so she could do every one of them. Erin had a great adventure at camp that year. She was looking forward to returning the next year.

At the end of the camp, I asked each of the campers what we could do to make camp more exciting and fun the following year. I expected most of them to say to let them stay up later or s'mores every night. When I asked Erin, she looked up and said, "Hot air balloons and race cars." (Those are the people I like to run with!) I told her I would probably be afraid of going up in a hot air balloon. Erin replied, "Don't worry. I'll go up with you." She passed on before we did manage to get hot air balloons at camp several years later.

Still, she was in my thoughts throughout the time I was in that hot air balloon in Kenya. At the end of that ride over the African Plains, I received a certificate indicating I had completed the balloon flight. I changed the name on the certificate to Erin's and sent it to her parents. I also explained to them that many more people from around the world, who had shared that experience with me, had been told of their beautiful daughter.

MOTIVATED BY LOVE

A mother once wrote an article that appeared in *Exceptional Parent* magazine that moved me. She compared having a child born with disability to having a change of itinerary for an exotic vacation. She thought she was going to Rome, but she landed in Holland instead. It was a beautiful metaphor. The mother loved her child just the same, even though her destination, as a parent, was not the one she had foreseen.

There's a certain courage in being the parent of a child with a disability. And there's a definite courage revealed in the children who have disabilities. I've also learned that you have to be courageous when you try to make life better for these children and their families. You have to allow your heart to be broken, to be cleaved, to wrap it around this mission.

You have to allow your heart to be broken, to be cleaved, to wrap it around this mission.

Faith is a big part of that journey for me. Living in faith is not just a matter of belief in God. It is also dependent upon how often you have experienced sacred, mystical, and magical moments that involve interacting with other people—truly encountering them and their needs.

Through the years, I've gotten better in my work with children, whether it's here in the United States or in other countries through Timmy Global Health. I've learned how to consider the climate, the politics, the culture, and the economics of different countries. All of those logistical difficulties are easier to overcome after we've had the experience of tackling them previously.

I've also come to realize there will never be a shortage of people in need. I once met with a professor of pediatric surgery when I had returned to Indianapolis after helping in another country.

He asked, "What are you doing now?"

I told him, and he said, "What a noble profession." I never heard anyone call this work "noble." He made me realize that I was committed to my work despite knowing I would never accomplish all of it. I just know that I will die trying.

I once told a friend, "I would give my life for these kids." Then, after a moment's reflection, I added, "I guess I already have."

COURAGEOUS CARE IN A BUREAUCRATIC JUNGLE

Healthcare workers need to be courageous and take risks. In 1990, David Carter, a respiratory therapist and hospital administrator, and Nancy McCurdy, a child life specialist, created CHAMP Camp. They recruited me to be the medical director. As we prepared to have the first week-long camp, here is the reality we considered, "We'll have twenty-six campers this year, most of whom cannot breathe on their own. Many of them are on ventilators, and the others are on machines that apply pressure into their airways, helping them to breathe. They've never been away from home without their parents ..." Still we decided, liability be damned, we were going to have the camp. We wanted to make life worth living for the campers. We had this crazy idea that to improve their quality of life, we must take risks, including liability risks.

I believe the children who are my patients have to have bragging rights. Medical records these days are created on computers. And they often don't include a detailed social history that outlines the patient's education, hobbies, and interests.

I ask my patients, "What's something outrageous you've always wanted to do, something that seems impossible?" My goal is to make that wish happen for them. They don't know it, but I record those wishes in their charts and in my heart, and we start our movement in that direction.

Some of the ideas for helping them live their dreams have come from some unique

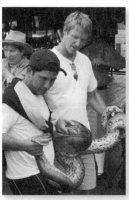

opportunities. In 2005, a group of us floated down the Rio Negro in Brazil on a houseboat, providing medical care. Some of the villagers caught an anaconda and said, "Here, hold this, and get a photo." I've always dreamed of "bagging and tagging"

How do we take the jungle to the hospital?

animals in the rainforest, so it seemed like a cool idea—until the giant snake wrapped around my left wrist. For a while, I was sure I would never get my hand back. You've heard the old adage, "meaner than a snake." This one fit that description. It became a point of concern as to how we were going to get it off me without anybody getting bitten. Eventually, the villagers helped free me from the sixteen-foot-long anaconda.

That experience gave me an idea. We started a program with the help of my buddy Tony who owned a pet shop. He had a fifteen-foot-long python, a six-foot-long alligator, and some other cool animals we brought to the hospital so the children could experience them. Risk was involved, but we took every precaution, including taping the alligator's mouth shut. When the kids got out of the hospital and went back to school, people would ask them, "Where have you been for six weeks?" They could reply, "Well, I was taming an alligator. I had a tarantula crawling on my head. I have photos of myself with scorpions." Life in the hospital needs to be beyond normal so returning to school will feel like a walk in the park.

THE GIFT OF THE IMPOSSIBLE

We also have to be supportive. Kathy has a disease that affects the cartilage, tendons, and ligaments. When I met her, she was one of our CHAMP campers. Kathy has to live on a ventilator at night, but she's still lived a full life. In high school, she was a straight-A student. Yet, Kathy's vocational rehabilitation counselor told her, "You're so disabled you should either get a job at McDonald's or learn to do handicrafts at home." Kathy didn't accept that advice. Instead, she went to college, where she made the dean's list every semester. She also volunteered on nine Timmy trips to seven different countries. We took her ventilator with us, along with Ambu bags to manually push air into her lungs, in case we didn't have electricity and needed to bag her at night. Fortunately, it all worked out. She was courageous at every turn. The patients in our clinics were inspired by her presence and her efforts. We were too.

During my time in India, two surgeons and I did simple procedures on the legs of children so they could stand up, walk, and talk to people face to face. It made a big difference in other ways for these children, too. It removed the stigma of the disability, making it possible for these children to go to school and even one day to marry. When we returned from India, the two surgeons who accompanied me got asked the same question I did, "How successful was your trip? How many surgeries did you do?"

"It was very successful. We did twenty-six surgeries," I would say. Then I would add, "We've only got about three million to go."

We have to live in the belief that each of those twenty-six children might reach twenty-six others, and those twenty-six others might touch twenty-six more. I came back to this country and talked to rooms filled with more than twenty-six people, sometimes hundreds or thousands. I continue to talk to people, inviting them to be part of this effort. It's the way the ripple effect that Mother Teresa always talked about becomes real. The number of people helping others gets higher and higher, and that's how we heal our world.

To remind myself to encourage others to join me and get involved in helping others, I kept a quote from Mother Teresa taped to my mirror: "It's not my job to be successful. It is my job to be faithful."

CHAPTER 6

Be Compassionate

C ompassion literally means "to suffer with." Henri Nouwen and other writers have described it as seeing someone suffering and having the willingness to share and experience that suffering with them. I also like the phrase, "Step into the fire"—to share someone's pain, to try to alleviate it.

I believe we are wired to be compassionate. Courtney is a perfect example of this human trait. She and two other eight-year-old girls came up to me after one of my talks.

"I found this baby bird in the grass. It had fallen out of its nest," she said to me as she rocked side to side on her feet, pushing her wire-rim glasses back onto her nose. "There was no mother to protect it. I tried to feed him some worms, and he didn't eat them. And then I tried to feed him some bread. And he didn't eat that. So I hid him in the high grass so that the cat wouldn't get him. And then I stayed with him until he flew back to heaven."

That's what it means to be compassionate.

There is a beautiful Sanskrit word, *Karuna*, that means "sharing, removing and transforming suffering." If you are caring enough to meet another living being in

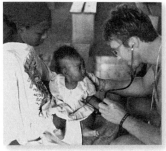

Mutual Healing

need and you alleviate that need, you have gone from compassion to Karuna. Healing is a mutual experience, and compassion is communal. One of my favorite authors, Joseph Girzone, distinguished between solidarity and charity. He described charity as throwing money into the panhandler's cup as one walks by and solidarity as taking a knee

> *Healing is a mutual experience, and compassion is communal.*

next to that same individual and getting to know his story. How is it possible for us to have compassion for others when we have not truly encountered them? How is it possible for us to move to Karuna without really knowing the person we are encountering? As I tell my political friends, "You cannot fix these problems by throwing money at them. You fix these problems by throwing good people at them!"

WHAT IS THE VALUE OF A HUMAN LIFE?

When I was in Ecuador several years ago, my clinic was a chair under the swing set on a school playground. After finishing the morning session, I ran to grab something to eat. When I returned, there was an adorable little boy leaning on the chair where I had been sitting. I said, "Hola!" He replied, "Hola!" and thrust his hand up to shake mine. His dad called him by name, and Luis returned to his place in the line of children to be examined by me.

Most of the children I evaluated were healthy. Some had minor problems such as a headache or a fungal infection. When Luis stepped forward with his dad, I learned that Luis was four years old, not two or three as I had thought due to his small stature.

You cannot fix these problems by throwing money at them. You fix these problems by throwing good people at them!

His father asked, "Do you have medicine for a cough and leg pain?"

I said, "Yes, but let me just take a quick listen to your son."

I set the stethoscope on his chest, which was heaving. He had what's called a "thrill," a rumbling in the chest caused by violent movement of the blood due to a congenital heart problem. I could hear a loud heart murmur through the stethoscope.

"Are you aware that Luis has heart disease?" I asked his father.

"Si, yes, I know this," his father said. "But I have four other children, and I only make $1,500 a year, and the heart surgery is $7,000 US dollars, so I can't afford it."

Luis' father understood that his son would lag behind the other children, but he did not understand that Luis would die if he did not have surgery.

During that clinic, there were three young college students seeing patients with me. I instructed them to listen to Luis' heart through the stethoscope. After they listened, I asked, "What do you think? Is he worth $7,000?"

"Dr. Chuck, I can't believe you would even say that!" one young lady exclaimed.

"Well, you understand this isn't a hypothetical situation," I said. "We're not sitting in a classroom talking about it. This isn't a debate on health economics and inequalities. We have the means to save a child's life. What is that worth to each of us?"

In my mind, I had already calculated that I didn't need to lease a new car the following year. I could get by with less, and we could save this child's life for $7,000. How could we not? At the same time, I wanted the students to think about how much they were willing to give up. Would they give up a full semester of college? What if they fell a semester behind on getting their bachelor's degree, but they saved a life? What was that worth?

They decided Luis was certainly worth $7,000.

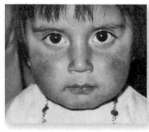

Primary Diagnosis: C.U.T.E.

I could have written a check to make it happen, but I learned from some great heroes of mine to sometimes do things based on faith. Instead, we shared this opportunity. The students took pictures of Luis and went back to their communities. They collected money in front of grocery stores. They asked people to donate their change. Hundreds of people contributed to saving that little boy's life.

We negotiated a deal with cardiovascular surgeons at the hospital on the north side of Quito, Ecuador. For $1,700, Luis received life-saving heart surgery. He now has a normal life expectancy. That same surgery would've cost about $180,000 in the United States.

Ultimately, we all must decide, "What is the value of each human life?" We all like to think we are not biased or prejudiced. The Bible says we are all created in God's image. We all tend to *create our God* in our own image. If we are vindictive, angry, and bitter, that's what our God looks like. If we're loving and forgiving, our image of God is much more like that of Jesus.

OUR HANDS

I have a sketch of Mother Teresa holding a baby to her face. The picture has always meant a lot to me because I used to make rounds on babies from the neonatal

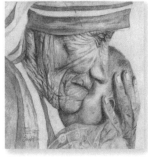

intensive care unit. The babies were surrounded by technology. Tubes went into different parts of their bodies.

Sketch of Mother Teresa
by Scarlet Cramer

They were attached to monitors. Usually, there wasn't much medical treatment we needed to provide. Surviving pre-term delivery takes time, nutrition, growth, and development. Still, I listened to their hearts, checked their lungs, and examined them for potential problems. There was also one other thing I did, a ritual that wasn't part of my medical training. I leaned my head down, placed my face against the babies' faces, cupped their heads, and whispered to them, "God loves you, and so do I." I felt technology wasn't allowing the human touch these children needed, because it was almost impossible to pick them up, cuddle them, or hold them. I tell parents how important it is for their child to feel their presence, to hear their voices, to experience their touch.

When the hospice program began at our children's hospital, mysterious things started happening. I'm no poet, but I started waking up in the middle of the night, writing entire poems in the notepad

> *God loves you, and so do I.*

beside my bed. The poems expressed the love and healing inspired by our little gurus in our sacred hospital setting.

The healing power of our hands was revealed through a baby named Chelsea. She was five months old when I stopped into her hospital room to evaluate her one morning. She had a metabolic disorder, and we didn't expect her to live beyond eight months of age. During my visit, I talked to Chelsea's mom. As I turned to leave, I noticed a black-and-white photograph on the wall. A friend of the family, a professional photographer, had taken a photo of the hands of each family member stacked atop each other. Chelsea's dad's hand was on the bottom. Mom's hand was on top of his. The hand of their three-year-old daughter rested on mom's hand. And Chelsea's small hand was on top of her sister's. It was a beautiful picture.

Amazingly, I had transcribed a poem a few nights earlier focusing on Chelsea's hands. When I saw the picture, I turned to Chelsea's mom and said, "I think I have something that belongs to you." I returned to her room later with the poem I had written down in the middle of the night earlier that week.

Even in the most difficult times, and maybe especially during those times, our compassion reveals our true spiritual connection.

CHAPTER 7

Be Ordinary

I believed there was no way I could ever do what Mother Teresa and the Missionaries of Charities did in India. I thought they were extraordinary. Yet when I worked with them in Calcutta, I found—and I mean this with the utmost respect—that they were ordinary people. However, they had an extraordinary mission.

That's the example we need to follow in our work: Even though we are ordinary, we can do the extraordinary.

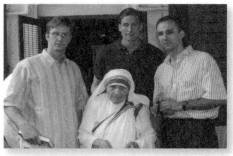

Mother Teresa was very short in stature, but she had a much larger presence.

Mother Teresa was very short in stature, but she had a much larger presence. You know that saying about how a moth is drawn to a flame? That's the impact Mother Teresa had on people. No one wanted to leave her presence. In fact, it was as if we were disoriented when we actually met with her. When a priest announced it was time to depart, all of us were bumping into each other, moving about. But, it was clear, none of us were actually leaving her sphere. I finally grabbed her hands and bowed and kissed them. Everyone in the room followed suit.

If you are exemplary, you are setting an example that can be followed.

When I returned from meeting with Mother Teresa, I started telling people to be ordinary. The word "exemplary" often brings to mind "remarkable". If you are exemplary, you are setting an example that can be followed. I don't want the young people who volunteer at Timmy Global Health to think they can't do what doctors and nurses do. Our teams sometimes perform surgeries when we visit other countries, but the work itself is about simple compassion. And that's where we can all do the extraordinary. By stressing that ordinary yet meaningful nature of the work, our volunteers can make a bigger difference than just one person could.

Student volunteers at Timmy Global Health can come with me to serve in countries around the world. We will put them safely in environments where they can make a difference, hold or heal someone and create a positive impact—without any special training.

Volunteers who work with us in these impoverished places discover they have something to offer by being present in the lives of people in need. All of us have an inherent need to be heard, so as healers we need to train ourselves to listen and let individuals tell their stories. Consider how much better those individuals feel by just sharing the struggles they face with someone who cares to listen.

I pray my students hear: "I prayed and God sent you." "You're a godsend." "You're an angel who came to relieve my suffering." "You saved my life!"

Kindness is a gift anyone can give. Usually, the challenges we face are just based on logistics. How do we get the child to where the care is?

> *As healers we need to train ourselves to listen.*

Or how do we get the care to where the child is? I don't have all the skills these children need to be healed or maybe even cured, but I certainly have resources. Being aware of those resources—and understanding what I know and what I don't know—I determine whom to turn to and how to appeal to them to see if they can deliver what's necessary for a child in need.

It all comes back to realizing that you're an ordinary person with an extraordinary mission that only you are able to fulfill. Our missions are uniquely tailored for each of us, depending on where we are located and what we can do to help other people.

I stress three qualities needed to provide help to people: be flexible, be considerate, and have a sense of humor. We have to stay hopeful and avoid becoming cynical or pessimistic. Keeping hopeful is hard to do in our healthcare system in the United States. I look forward to a day when we spend more time with our patients than with the administrative tasks. We've reached a point in this country where it's not about quality care; it's about documenting that you performed quality care. Whether you did or not is insignificant. Still, we healers strive to promote providing that quality care.

There's an honor—the Gold Humanism Honor Society Award—that is given to some medical students. The award was established by a pediatric neurologist who wanted to stress to young doctors the importance of compassion and bedside manner—qualities often not cultivated in our healthcare system. The Gold Humanism Honor Society Award is now presented to

You're an ordinary person with an extraordinary mission.

medical students and doctors who are not only learned professionals but also compassionate caregivers. Nominations for the award are made by patients, doctors, and fellow students. I'm always pleased when a volunteer for Timmy Global Health receives this honor and many have. I was honored to speak at the induction ceremony at our medical school in the past, as so many of our Timmies had received the award.

I witnessed this kind of extraordinary compassion while working with Mother Teresa when we went into the Missionaries of Charity homes. Those receiving care were essentially abandoned souls who had been rescued from trash piles or found lying in the streets. In India, Haiti, and other countries, it isn't uncommon to see people of all ages, including children, discarded as if they're rubbish. Babies and toddlers are left on doorsteps or in gutters, where they are rescued and cared for by these nuns. What the sisters provide is simple care. It usually isn't complex medical care. Mostly, it's bathing, feeding and, most importantly, holding the children who desperately need human touch.

Right after I met Mother Teresa in Calcutta in 1997, I walked across the courtyard into the orphanage called *Shishu Bhavan*, "The Home of the Little Ones." They asked me to remove my shoes, and I tiptoed between all of the children. There were babies and toddlers all over the floor and maybe eight people to take care of them. They prayed for people to show up, to help them with the children. And we, and others, did. I don't know what drew me, but there was this one baby that caught my attention. When I knelt to pick her up, another little girl came running through the other children and held onto my leg. All of a sudden, there was a migration of children toward me from around the room.

In that moment, what I now call *the* moment, I realized that we are much larger spiritually than the bodies we occupy. In fact, I tell our volunteers, "We can't give you an out-of-body experience, but we will give you a bigger-than-body experience." We are part of something bigger, the interconnectedness of all human beings. When all dimensions come together at the right time, in the right place, with the right motive, all the prepara-

> *We are much larger spiritually than the bodies we occupy.*

tion and resources intersect in that moment. When I go into these places, I don't always speak these people's languages. But I don't fear these people. I love to pick up the children and have them run their hands over my face—to show them that even though our skin colors are different, the feel of the skin is the same.

That's why I tell people, "If you ever held somebody, if you ever touched somebody, you have something to offer. We all have the capacity to heal another person."

I never want my patients or their families to feel they cannot approach me. It's imperative that families feel comfortable asking me questions so I can give the best care and educate them for the best possible outcomes for their children. I need to be able to answer their questions in plain, simple English. It's important to make sure the child's treatment options are clearly understood.

> *If you ever held somebody, if you ever touched somebody, you have something to offer. We all have the capacity to heal another person.*

Working in a children's hospital, we need to remind ourselves the hospital exists for the children, not for us. We just happen to be the ones blessed to care for the children. My focus is to offer hope and comfort to the children and their families. Sometimes, I do that in small and unusual ways. If I wear a tie around the children's hospital, it's usually a SpongeBob SquarePants tie.

I have a tie with an image of the game of Operation. I've also worn Christmas ties that play music or stick-on ties.

As I hurry through the waiting areas outside surgical suites, I see parents waiting for children who are in surgeries behind closed doors. They are anxious and concerned. Many of them are praying. But when I walk through and they look up to see one of those ties, even in those circumstances, it brings smiles to their faces. The ties are familiar, and the familiar gives people comfort. I keep that in mind every morning when I get dressed for work. That's why I sometimes wear those ties.

CHAPTER 8

Be True

I f we are going to serve youth, we need to trust them and believe in their ability to make a difference. That's why I asked David to join the board of directors of Timmy Global Health when he was eleven. David has cerebral palsy. He is also very bright and a great person to have along on our trips to other countries. On one occasion, he joined me in Ecuador. At the time, he wore braces on his legs. During that trip, a mother asked me, "My son, will he ever walk?"

"Yes, he will," I told her, but she couldn't believe it. So I added, "We need a little bit of medication, and we'll get him some braces—just a minute." I yelled into the hallway for David. David walked in, and I asked him to pull up his pant legs. When she saw David, the mother regained hope. She started to believe that her two-year-old son would one day walk again. She even talked about him visiting another country someday. As tears flowed down her cheeks, her son reached up and gently brushed them away.

Margie Luna is another young person who made an incredible difference. After returning from a trip to India in 1997, I ran down the hallway of the children's hospital in Indianapolis, heading for the clinic, trying to get caught up on my work. That's when I noticed a beautiful, bald-headed, teenaged girl anchored to an IV pole in the cancer clinic. As I rushed by, I smiled, said hello, and gave a brief wave. I heard a nurse yell, "Margie, that's the doctor that met Mother Teresa." Margie leapt from her chair, snatched her IV pole, and ran me down. When she reached me, she grabbed my arm. She said, "Please, Dr. Chuck, tell me about meeting with Mother Teresa."

I told her about the moment I met Mother and the work we were doing in India. I also gave her a rosary that had been blessed by Mother Teresa. Margie was thrilled. Even more, she was excited about the help we were giving to the people there. She said she wanted to help, too. She opted to forego her original wish, a Versace gown for the prom that Indiana Children's Wish Fund was to purchase, to go to India. We became great friends. Margie taught me what it feels like to love a daughter.

Margie began pressuring me to take her to India so she could care for the children with Mother Teresa. So I talked to her cancer doctor, and we monitored her blood counts to see if that would be a possibility. None of that mattered to Margie. She felt we should proceed with the trip regardless of her condition. She even sent me a letter encouraging me to arrange her trip the last week of November in 1997. The letter stated, "Dr. Chuck…Please, please, please (Imagine my please face here) can I go to India to work for the missionaries of charity? I feel it's my calling to help little children like Mother Teresa did."

We weren't able to go to India until February of 1998. Mother Teresa had passed over on September 5, 1997, but Margie visited her tomb, and one of the sisters gave Margie a rose from Mother's memorial. The trip was a great spiritual experience for Margie. As she spent time with the children in the orphanage, Margie's radiance was so obvious. She knew this was part of what she was here on Earth to do.

When we returned to Indianapolis, 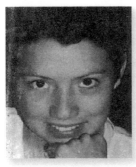 she continued her work generating love among people at her high school, the community, and the state. Margie's beautiful spirit radiated universally. Unfortunately, her cancer ulti-

Margie

mately returned. We knew her time was limited. I still remember the day we all came to the hospital to meet with Margie as she received the news. It was so tearful and sad. I couldn't talk with Margie at that time about the likelihood of her not being cured. As for Margie, she felt she had more work to do here on Earth.

Later that day, I went to her home. We cried, hugged, and talked about how difficult it was to face the cancer again. She had opted for minimal treatment, but there was little hope for a cure. Margie said, "I promise you, Dr. Chuck, if I die, I will be your guardian angel." In return, I promised her that we would take care of the children in Ecuador, where Margie had lived the first four years of her life.

Margie passed over in August of 1998. I still carry the above picture. I also carry with me one important lesson from Margie: Speak the truth, and follow through. Margie was a great example of being true.

A year from the day of Margie's death, I attended a memorial service for Margie in Quito, Ecuador. I met the priest who celebrated the mass, Padre Carollo. People called him "the Mother Teresa of Ecuador." We had a great talk, and he took me to see the work he was doing. I thought, *This is how we make this happen, what we promised Margie we'd do.* We joined forces with Padre Carollo's Tierra Nueva Foundation to build a hospital and do regularly scheduled clinics in the barrios. It took years to finish the Un Canto de la Vida Hospital (the Song of Life Hospital). The original cost estimate to build the hospital was per bed, or $500,000. But the economy collapsed in Ecuador in 2000, and the country switched to the US dollar. When Padre Carollo originally took me to the site of the hospital, he explained that the foundation had $100,000. So they bought the land, built the foundation, put in the drainage, and fenced in the area. He said, "Now I pray". With that, I said, "Father, could you come to the US and be my CFO?" I liked the idea of him being my Chief financial officer, or perhaps my Chief faith

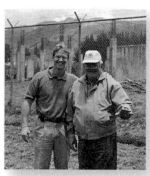

My CFO

officer. Ultimately, it cost $7 million to build a hospital with 139 beds. (Incidentally, it now costs approximately $2.6 to 3 million per bed to build hospitals in the United States.) Timmy Global Health now serves thirty-four communities in Ecuador in Margie's memory.

146

If you find people who affect you the way Margie affected me, and you make them a promise, see it through. People ask me, "You've worked in all these other countries. Why is Ecuador so important?" I answer, "My guardian angel is watching."

FRIENDS IN PREDICAMENTS

I used to host margarita nights for my patients who were twenty-one and older. Because we live in a litigious society, I was told, "If you're going to do that, you better document it." I had to prepare my defense if the authorities came after me. All of my twenty-one-and-older patients, most of whom had cerebral palsy, needed me to write them scripts stating they may go with their caregivers to have a drink. On the prescriptions for the supported living programs, I wrote, "Mindy may go out and have a drink."

We would go to a couple of restaurants known for the best margaritas. On occasion, I invited some of my friends who were not in the healthcare field. At the end of one night, a friend said, "It's awesome the way you treat them like they're normal." I replied, "They are. They're friends of mine who happen to be in predicaments." I'm happy to report we never had any legal problems with margarita nights. Lots of laughs; no lawsuits.

Still, there have often been other problems we've had to overcome. And many of the challenges are not related to age or impairment. Consider the story of Ethan. By the time he was five, he had survived about twenty-five brain surgeries—and

Medicaid had covered the cost of all of them. He also had a very large head with multiple deformities and disproportionately small extremities. Despite those challenges, Ethan loved exploring his world. He would roll and slide his head across the floor to get to books and toys. When it came time for Ethan to go to school, he needed battery-powered mobility. Yet, a Medicaid representative said, "No, he doesn't need a wheelchair." After covering the cost of twenty-five brain surgeries, I couldn't understand why Medicaid wouldn't help him now. It was absurd.

People have asked me, "Chuck you've worked in twenty-some other countries. How many languages do you speak?"

I usually say, "I'm fluent in two of them, English and vulgarity, but I'm trying to cut down on the second." After dealing with insurance companies, and some of the red tape that comes with getting my patients the care they need, it's often harder to use English than vulgarity.

When we talked with the Medicaid case management staff about Ethan, I exclaimed, "Are you kidding me? We came this far, and now we don't give him quality of life? That doesn't make sense!" But they wouldn't budge.

So I went to Eric, a buddy of mine. Eric was a young man with leukemia who had gone through chemotherapy, which had caused arthritis of his joints. Despite his challenges, he managed to get his bachelor's degree in engineering. I told Eric about Ethan and asked him to get some of his fellow students together to see if they could help. The students designed and built a prototype specifically for Ethan so

he could drive around—and to school—
in a modified toy Jeep. Ethan didn't get a
wheelchair; he got something a lot cooler.
It was the greatest gift anyone could have
given him. Ethan would burst out into a
belly laugh, pop that Jeep into gear, and
scream and laugh as he drove away.

Ethan is a good reminder that when
we start discussing public health issues,
economics, and cost efficiency in the
delivery of care, we have to keep our focus
on the value of the individual. When I
once went to the Dominican Republic,
a little boy was brought in to see me by
his mother. Jamison looked very sick. He
was jaundiced, he was bleeding from the
rectum, and he had a fever. I remember
evaluating him and thinking it could be
any number of life-threatening ailments. I
turned to the director of the mission and

said, "We need lab work. What would it cost to get all of these blood levels done?"

"$270," she answered.

"Okay, great. We'll give you that," I said.

"But we can feed all these kids for that much money for a month."

"Okay," I said. "We'll give you $540."

That's our approach at Timmy Global Health. We don't just advise people, wish them well, and then pray for them. We see it through. We make sure they get the transportation, the medications, the work-ups, and the surgeries they need.

If we minimize the value of an individual life, our organization is worthless. We lose the meaning of our work. $540 is not a huge sum. I look around a room, and between everyone in that room, I know together we can scratch up that sum.

CHAPTER 9

Be Selfless

I think of my life as a journey to becoming selfless. As with so many spiritual journeys, learning selflessness means trying to give as much of yourself as possible so you can relate to and respond to others. I realize I still have a way to go in this journey. Yet one of the lessons I've learned along the way is that patients need me to acknowledge them and speak directly. Concerned parents in the clinic pay far more attention to what you say to their children than what you say to them directly. Some of my patients have said about me, "He didn't come in and talk to my parents. He spoke to me. He got on the floor with me or sat in a chair next to my wheelchair. We were face to face."

The truth is, I've never given more than I've received in return. I love my job! I'm the caregiver of my spiritual leaders. Yet, because there are so many who are in need, it wears on me at times.

In 1999, when I met Padre Carollo in Ecuador, he confided, "Chuck, my life is not my own." I said, "Yes, Father. I know exactly what you mean." My mission was growing, and I was already at a point of no return, both locally and globally. Between my work at the local children's hospital in Indianapolis and my efforts in the developing world, it was clear there was no turning back.

I've had to remind people with whom I've worked in the past—both at the hospital and in the medical field in underserved countries—that we're in the business of helping others. Therefore, we will be inconvenienced. That's part of this calling. You're not always going to get requests for assistance or a need for an emergency response at convenient times, such as in the middle of the day. It might be late at night when you're trying to rest or take some time for yourself. You have to be willing to forgo personal comfort and many desires.

My professional commitment has been costly on many levels. I have struggled with my ability to commit to marriage and have my own family, but I have been consumed by my life's work up to this point. Loss has been a prominent feature in the history of people I've loved throughout my life, whether they were foster children, personal friends, or hospice patients. It has put some wear and tear on my heart.

When people talk to me about love, loss, pain, anguish, grief, and depression, I understand. I've been there. I'm keeping in touch regularly with a girl who has done some work with us in Ecuador. She's in high school, and she has volunteered to work with the poor in the Amazon rainforest. I didn't realize she was going through tough times. One day, I wanted to thank her for doing a good job in the clinic and went looking for her. Her father told me, "She's sitting out in front of the building." I went there and sat next to her. She was crying and very distraught. She was frustrated by her peers' lack of empathy. At the time, I was in an emotionally tough place, too—feeling despair and heartache over a recent breakup with my fiancée. As I sat with this girl in the rainforest, it was helpful and healing for both us to discuss compassion and meeting the needs of others.

At one point, I said, "You wouldn't know this, but I just lost the woman I thought I would marry. The reason you feel the way you do is because you're a sensitive soul. You care about the world and about the people in it. You will not go through this world without a lot of pain; you won't be unscathed. Because you do care and have compassion, when you finish high school and go on to nursing school, you're going to be an outstanding nurse. You will be an outstanding healer because of your ability to fully open yourself to these experiences and empathize with others."

ABILITY TO SEE BEYOND OUR OWN NEEDS

Jordan was a cute little guy who had the biggest brown eyes. He was diagnosed with spinal muscular atrophy, which is similar to Lou Gehrig's disease in children. Jordan drove a battery-powered wheelchair with a joystick. He once drew me a picture

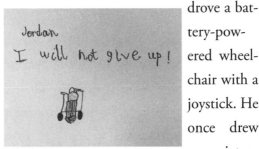

Drawing by Jordan

of himself walking in his rolling walker. On the paper, he wrote, "I will not give up!" When Jordan came to clinic one day, he was his usual lively, mischievous self. I was excited to tell him about the local Challenger Little League that would give all children, regardless of disability, an opportunity to play baseball. Because Jordan would soon be turning six, he was eligible to play in the league, which made him extremely excited. When I gave him information on how to register for the league, Jordan assured me he would have his paperwork filled out as soon as possible.

That night, I received a phone call from Jordan's father. He told me that Jordan was so excited when he got home that he told his dad he needed shorts, socks, pants, a hat, a T-shirt, and sweatbands for his arms. He also informed his father he would need cleats. As his dad was talking to me, he said, "You know, it never occurred to Jordan that he can't walk, let alone run."

On opening day of the baseball season, Jordan sat along the first base path in his battery-powered wheelchair. He had black marker under his eyes and wore new Nike cleats. He held his hat over his heart as "The Star Spangled Banner" was played. Although Jordan was described as a good kid, he did steal that day. He stole second base in his wheelchair.

Jordan was also a star off the field. Two years later, I received a phone call. I was asked if I would write a letter to Jordan's class, thanking them for what they had done for the children in the hospital. Jordan had gone to school and made this suggestion: Instead of the first-grade children buying gifts for each other that Christmas, they should pool their money and buy Christmas presents for the children who would be in Dr. Chuck's hospital during the Christmas holidays.

That was Jordan. He never gave up. Even more importantly, he kept giving of himself. His actions are a reminder to all of us: No matter our circumstances in life, we are all born to be healers.

NURTURING A GIVING SPIRIT

Mother Teresa once said, "We know only too well that what we are doing is nothing more than a drop in the ocean. But if the drop were not there, the ocean would be missing something."

I was deeply touched by my time with Mother Teresa, and I received pieces of her sari from the sisters after she passed over. When I received that gift, I also began to think about how I should share it. I went to a jeweler for help in designing and making silver pendants with the image of Mother Teresa and the logo of Timmy Global Health. And I checked with nuns and priests to make sure that creating the pendants would be allowable. On the back of these pendants is written, "…small things with great love." Mother used to say, "We can do no great things, only small things with great love." Inside each of these pendants is a thread from Mother's sari.

I give these pendants to people who are instrumental in our work at Timmy Global Health. They are presented as an award and a commitment, and I also hope that it serves as a reminder to each of them of the importance of this sacred mission and the need for it to be pure. Our individual works seem small, but they do create a ripple effect. I tell the recipients we're not going to clothe the naked with a single thread, but when all our threads are woven together, we will clothe them.

> *We're not going to clothe the naked with a single thread, but when all our threads are woven together, we will clothe them.*

That's our legacy. And Mother Teresa blesses our work. I have a letter from her stating that she does.

We have a spiritual commitment to see this through, to be as selfless as we can in helping others. This is my true calling. I also ask people to be who they were meant to be. I ask them to bring whatever gift they have and share it with others. I invite them to help heal this world. Timmy Global Health allows them that opportunity.

Years ago, I told the people who worked with Mother Teresa in India that if they would just put a roof over my head and feed me once a day, I'd stay there the rest of my life to take care of the kids. I don't think they took me seriously, but I meant it. In the years that followed, I often woke up in the middle of the night with ideas about how to help children in difficult circumstances. I wrote those ideas in a notebook. I constantly pondered how we could deliver medicine and supplies or build another school. Could we build a clinic? How often could we continue to assist patients in a certain country?

With those ideas and questions came a realization: I had to recruit more leaders and more healers, learn to delegate responsibilities to others, and take on a mentorship role with Timmy Global Health. I am happy to tell you the students and volunteers have never let me down. They respond with the greatest efforts. They're doing wonderful service for others around the globe. I believe in their creativity, their compassion, and their abilities. I admire their selflessness and passion. Our job is to gently guide the reins, to direct the efforts of the students, but we must never pull back on the reins.

CHAPTER 10

Be Humble

We all have different missions or callings in life. Humility is understanding that one person's mission is no more or less important than another's.

Still, in our American culture, we're often viewed and defined by what we do for a living or how much money we make. Some people respond differently to me when they learn that I'm a doctor. The point is that being a doctor is what I do. It's not *who* I am. Humility, or having a humble nature, is an expression of appreciation for the gifts you possess, what you've been given. There's no room in that definition for thinking you're more valuable than anyone else or having a haughty attitude about your talents. I firmly believe that your gifts and talents are meant to be shared with others while you're in this world. If you don't appreciate others' roles in this life as having the same importance as your own, then the community is weakened.

The Missionaries of Charity sisters once asked me if I wanted to meet the pope. I said, "No offense to the pope, but Mother Teresa is first on my list." I developed this great affinity for her after I read about her, her compassion, and her selfless approach of giving herself to others. It shaped how I viewed my life of faith and my philosophy of life.

I think Mother Teresa also challenged us to give more of what we have—our gifts—and to do it not only selflessly but tirelessly. When I once gave a lecture, I was introduced with the words, "Dr. Dietzen's tireless efforts to help the underserved..." I leaned over to a friend of mine who was sitting with me and said, "Actually, I'm exhausted."

I want to be wrung out when I leave this dimension. There's nothing better than to feel you have done everything you could to benefit others, that you have given every ounce of your physical and spiritual energy. I joke with my friends that I don't know if I'm going to get to do all of this cool stuff after I'm dead, so I want to pursue it all while I'm here. On occasion, I just have to call timeout and leave the arena. I take time for myself when I play sports, fish, wander, or climb mountains. I've even been known to go dog sledding. I also become re-energized by praying and taking time to think about life. After I recharge, I'm ready for more. Still, it is only when I encounter the next child in need that the energy and spirit fully return.

THE POPE MEETS JOE

In 2001, I was granted an audience with Pope John Paul II. Among the many qualities I admire about him are the number of Jewish friendships he maintained and the lives he helped preserve throughout World War II. I enjoyed studying his face when he prayed. He is another one of my spiritual heavyweights, a list that includes the Dalai Lama, Thich Nhat Hanh, and Mother Teresa. When I was invited to meet with Pope John Paul II, I asked one of my patients, Joe, to go with me. His trip was eventually made possible by the Indiana Children's Wish Fund.

Joe is a young man who was in a sledding accident. He went headfirst into a tree. It fractured his neck and left him quadriplegic. He underwent his rehabilitation in our hospital. During a clinic visit, he asked me, "Do you think the foundation would grant my wish to go see the Roman ruins in Italy?"

"Well, I think they probably would," I said. "But I've got a question for you. How would you like to meet the pope while you're there?"

"If it was anybody but you asking, I'd think you were bullshitting me," Joe responded.

"Well, I've been told I'm going to be granted an audience with him," I said. "Why don't you go with me? We'll go over and do it all in one trip."

The trip was Joe's first in a plane. He's about six feet four inches tall and weighs 220 pounds—a big guy. His family and I had to carry him onto the plane in a sheet sling, put him in a seat, and secure him with a strap. We had long flights with connections, to and from Rome. Through it all, Joe was awesome. So was our time in Rome.

I knew we were being granted an audience with the pope, but we weren't sure which day. It finally happened on my birthday. We went to the general audience, where the pope had an outdoor blessing, which he did in several different languages. I took Joe in his chair and pushed him up the long incline to where the pope stood.

They lined all of us up, and the pope blessed each one of us. The following day, we had another audience with him, in the papal palace. Despite his station in the Catholic Church, Pope John Paul II was very approachable. That impressed me. I hope that I will always be approachable and that other people will always feel they can come to me when they are in need. I would hate to get to a point where people had to prevent others from having access to me.

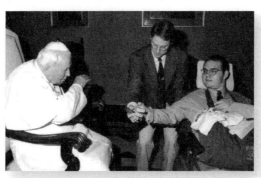

The pope got to meet Joe.

We have photos of both meetings with the pope. Visitors don't shoot their own photographs, because the Vatican has its own photographer. When I got back to my clinic, someone said, "Let me see this photo. I've been hearing so much about it." I showed this picture of Joe and me in front of Pope John Paul II. Many people told me, "I think it's great Joe got to meet the Pope." I said, "I think it's great the pope got to meet Joe."

Joe has a reclining wheelchair because of his inability to move his arms and legs. On occasion, if his blood pressure drops too low, you can release the chair and lay him back. When we went to the Sistine Chapel, people were asked not to lie on the floor to look at the ceiling. We tilted Joe back in his chair, and he had the ultimate view as we rolled him through Michelangelo's masterpiece.

Joe is a work of art himself. He's a phenomenal, spiritual being. He has a wonderful heart, and he's accomplished great things, including graduating from college. He also has made a positive impact on others' lives. At first, the nurses were concerned about Joe because he wasn't "depressed enough" after he became quadriplegic. I said, "Have you spent time talking with him? He's a remarkable young man. He sees meaning in everything that has happened to him."

We call him, "Super Joe." That's now his email address. He was called Super Joe by some people in Kenya because he helped them develop an agricultural program for kids at an orphanage there. From his home office, Joe was able to gather and forward information from Purdue University's School of Agriculture to a New Zealander taking care of several children in Kenya. The New Zealander needed agricultural data to provide enough food for the orphans. The program was successful, and the orphaned Kenyan children and their caregivers were thankful for Joe's hard work.

TRYING TO HELP THE WORLD

For much of my medical career, I was so consumed by my work that I couldn't sleep at night. The world was full of children who were suffering;

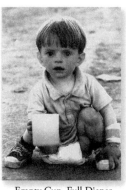

Empty Cup, Full Diaper

children at risk; children without adequate nutrition, education, shelter or healthcare. It was torturous trying to sleep, knowing bad things were happening to kids in all the locations I visited worldwide. I felt the need to gather as many resources as possible in the United States and return to them.

Disposable diapers are an expensive commodity. In one Kosovar refugee camp, each child was allotted one diaper per day, as it was not only difficult to obtain the diapers but to dispose of them properly. Controlling diarrheal diseases is a great concern when there are so many children on just a few acres of land. This photo was taken toward the end of the day when we had distributed all of the food. By dusk, the cup was empty but the diaper was full.

Later, working in a children's hospital in El Salvador, I witnessed mothers wringing out wet diapers to put them back on their children. I discovered that each diaper costs $1. These families were living on an income of $5 per day. This prompted us to initiate a diaper drive here in Central Indiana that allowed us to send five thousand diapers to that hospital. I used to joke that I had to get a larger globe because my small globe deceived me into believing I could reach every one of these kids in every place on Earth. Ultimately, what I had to do was engage more students for Timmy Global Health and introduce them to the philosophy that all these children have great value and need our assistance. I tell the high school and college students, "I am not here to recruit followers. I am here to recruit leaders."

We need students to help heal the world. I believe that if we invite them to be a part of our efforts to help children, they will be able to discern what they should do with their futures, and they will also help us provide a healing presence immediately.

> *I am not here to recruit followers.*
> *I am here to recruit leaders.*

"I need you, and I need you now," I tell students. "I don't want to wait for you to get a degree. We already have much that needs to be done, and you have the skills to help us."

That recruitment approach has allowed me to get some sleep. It has also allowed Timmy Global Health to create a mass movement of volunteers—mostly students, with big hearts and bright minds—to start creating change.

WORLDWIDE CHANGE STARTS ONE STUDENT AT A TIME

In recent years, people have said to me, "You must be very, very proud of Timmy's growth." I've replied, "I'm not proud of what I've done with Timmy Global Health, but I am extremely proud of what these young students—the high-school, college, and even kindergarten students—have done to help us heal the world. I'm very proud of them."

I often tell parents of Timmy volunteers, "I couldn't love your kids more, unless they were my own sons and daughters." I always thank the parents for instilling in their sons and daughters values we can nurture.

In founding and helping to build Timmy, I have prayed regularly, and I have

> *I couldn't love your kids more, unless they were my own sons and daughters.*

made it my life's commitment to provide accessible, quality healthcare for all. I believe this is what God wants from me, so this is how I will live my life—taking care of children. I used to think I would be married by the age of twenty-five and have eight kids. My life hasn't always gone the way I expected it, which has served to keep me humble and focused on my goal of building a better world for our children.

FINDING SUCCESS IN HUMBLE CIRCUMSTANCES

Kiley is a beautiful, radiant soul who happens to have cerebral palsy. She traveled to Ecuador with me to heal others recently. Cerebral palsy affects the right side of her body, so her right arm and leg don't work so well. She was pretty weak and spastic on that side when we first met. At the time, I thought, *I hope no one's teasing her at school.* I used to talk to her parents about that— and how bad it would look if Dr. Chuck had to show up on the playground to kick some bully's butt.

I met Kiley when she was two years old. I remember when she came down the clinic hallway, the whole place lit up. I hugged her and whispered, "Kiley, don't tell the others, but you're my favorite patient." I might have said that to a couple of other patients through the years, but we joke about it. She still sends me cards, which say, "Don't tell the others, but you're my favorite doctor."

It breaks my heart to think somebody might pick on these kids, but Kiley taught me a valuable lesson. I was still very involved

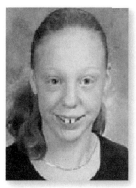

in football and rugby then. I'd take time away from the hospital to go play sports. Kiley was about ten years old when I returned from one of those trips. She had been

"Guess what, Dr. Chuck, I don't get last anymore!"

running track and playing soccer. Imagine doing that when one of your arms and one of your legs don't work well. I would probably run the hundred-meter event because that race is over quickly. Not Kiley. She ran the quarter mile and half mile.

"How are things going? Are you still doing sports?" I asked.

"Great," she said. "I'm still playing soccer."

"Aren't you running track?"

"Oh yeah. And guess what, Dr. Chuck, I don't get last anymore!"

That's the lesson I learn from these kids. Their courage keeps me humble and makes me want to do all I can for them. It's fun to have them as teammates in the game of life. Now, I don't have to win … I'm just content to be a participant on the field and cheerleader for my heroes!

CHAPTER 11

Be Hopeful

We all have hopes. All parents hope their children will be born healthy. A child may hope to become a dancer, an athlete, a doctor, a musician— the possibilities are endless.

Being hopeful means you've had time to prepare for what's ahead, so you've envisioned the possibilities. You have also committed yourself to making them happen. You can have a vision if you allow yourself to have one. You need to know what you know and know what you don't know to be a good healer. If you know what you don't know, you can be more resourceful.

> *You need to know what you know and know what you don't know to be a good healer.*

I always tell the doctors I train, "Being a great doctor isn't just a matter of being knowledgeable. Med school made me more knowledgeable, but my patients made me wiser." Because of my patients, I have often experienced a similar situation

> *Med school made me more knowledgeable, but my patients made me wiser.*

previously. I know where I can track down the resources and relevant information to shed light on certain circumstances. Sometimes, I know someone who can solve a dilemma. Always, I'm focused on giving my patients hope.

I once shot a photo of a little girl with her mother in Haiti that was published in a day planner. In the photo, they are sitting in line, waiting to be seen in the clinic. The

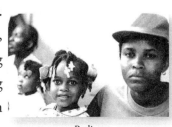

Radiance

little girl's eyes are simply radiant. In fact, the photograph is titled "Radiance." The eyes of the mother reflect a different perspective. Someone described the mother's eyes as "vacant." They look hopeless. The spirit is no longer present in her eyes. When I share that photo, I challenge people, "How do we keep the little girl's eyes from becoming her mother's eyes?" Our job is to make sure the radiance remains throughout her life, that she has a vision, that dreams are possible for her.

I'm concerned about our world. We're not doing a good enough job protecting and healing our children so they can grow up safe, have dreams, and fulfill their destinies. Whether they have unlimited abilities or disabilities is insignificant. Are they growing spiritually? Are they getting the nutrition they need? Are they allowed a time of innocence? Do they have access to a good education? Are they safe—protected from the climate, natural disasters, and war? So many children are in war zones.

How do we protect children? Healthcare is my toehold of hope. It gets my foot in the door in many regions of the world. Beyond medical care, other factors

> *Our job is to make sure the radiance remains throughout her life.*

contribute to public health issues, such as infrastructure. People say, "Well, you're a pediatric rehab doc. Why are you building schools? Why are you so concerned about good roads?" Good infrastructure can prevent bad things from happening to kids. It is preventative medicine. If four children come to the clinic in Haiti with broken or sprained ankles from stepping in a pothole, I will treat the children, and then I will go and fill in the pothole. As the Minister of Health for Estonia once said to me, "My problem is I'm down river pulling people out of the water. I need to be up river keeping them from jumping in."

These are some of the many obstacles that must be addressed when you're trying to make sure you maintain the radiance in a little girl's eyes—when you're trying to ensure she remains hopeful about some sort of future for herself, her family, and her community.

HOPE DESPITE DISABILITY

Mary was twenty-one months old when I saw her in the clinic. She had tetramelia, which is the absence of both arms and legs at birth. She was a beautiful little girl who rolled about the room so that she could explore. As I held a picture book for her, she scanned it with her radiant eyes. Once she completed her examination of the pages, she leaned forward and turned the next page with her tongue. Her incredible determination brought tears to all of the eyes in the room.

Hope can surface when tragedy strikes. Leo was a high-school kid with a nose for trouble. He'd been suspended from school for selling drugs. Despite being on probation and restricted from certain locations, Leo went with his friend to see a girl they both knew. They thought it would be funny to take an empty pistol, put it in Leo's mouth, and pull the trigger. But there happened to be a bullet in the chamber. He was shot in the brain stem.

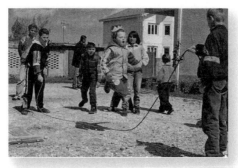

Take time to celebrate.

The accident made him quadriplegic. It also made him dependent on a ventilator to breathe. When he came to our hospital for rehabilitation, a nurse said to me, "Dr. Chuck, if this guy were not quadriplegic and could use his arms, I'm sure he would kill himself." I, too, thought he probably would commit suicide.

There was a bad snowstorm one day. As we looked at the snow, we had an idea that would give Leo hope and that made us say, "Liability be damned!" I have photos of this moment, and I describe it in my talks. I preface the story by saying, "If we have any risk management people in here, they might not want to hear this story." We took Leo off the vent and lifted him from his hospital bed. We put him on one of the mats from the gymnasium, and we pulled him outdoors into the snow.

We took Leo off his ventilator and dragged him around on a mat through the snow. One of the therapists sat on the mat holding him and bagging him with an Ambu bag, doing his breaths for him.

Big risk. If anything went wrong there, we would have all been at fault. After the ride, we took him back into the hospital and put him back in his bed. He turned a corner. He began to see there was still some potential for joy, even though he was totally quadriplegic.

Leo could still talk with the ventilator blowing air into his lungs. He had a wonderful mind and a loving heart. He was very bright. He and I sat down one day, and we talked. He looked at me and said, "Dr. Chuck, you wouldn't have liked who I used to be."

Later, I contacted officials at his school.

"He needs to go back to school," I said.

"No, he's not welcome here," they said. "He's nothing but trouble."

"I think he has a different perspective on life now," I said.

Leo was a remarkable person. He ended up with a retainer switch in the roof of his mouth so he could drive his wheelchair. He went to college after finishing high school to study psychology so he could work with troubled youth. I couldn't think of a better example of someone who could work with troubled youth than Leo. He just needed encouragement to understand that life's difficult experiences equip you to give hope to other people. None of us could reach that particular population like Leo could.

> *Difficult experiences equip you to give hope to other people.*

HOPE IS EVERYWHERE

There is hope even in death. That was a lesson I had to learn through experience. I wondered how I was going to survive children dying. How would I find hope in those situations? Some of the children and adults I worked with had died and been resuscitated. Their reports and the research on near-death experiences revealed to me that death wasn't something to fear and, in fact, they looked forward to returning to life after death. Their near-death experiences were comfortable, peaceful. They described them as incredible homecomings.

At the age of nine, my patient Jacob came back from clinical death. He had suffered a large hemorrhage into the brain. After recovering from the coma, he sat stooped in his wheelchair, a feeding tube in his nose, multiple staples in his scalp over the surgical site. When he discovered that there was a chapel in our hospital, he said, "I need to go pray." His mother, father, and 10 ten-year-old sister sat with him for several minutes, as he bowed his head and leaned forward in the wheelchair. His mother said they got antsy, and finally, his sister said, "Jacob! Jacob!" in an effort to awaken him. Without lifting his head, he said, "Shhh... I'm asking God into my heart."

> *I have never heard more people say, "God bless you," without anyone sneezing.*

Eventually, Jacob informed us, "I died, but I met Jesus." He hugged me and told me it wasn't time for me to die."

I think about Jacob a lot. If he

found peace even in the face of death, if he could find death to be healing, how can we not be more hopeful?

Despite all the sickness and trauma in the world, life goes on. As most people live their lives and plan their futures, people who are diagnosed as "terminally ill" feel they lose those years of their lives when they are battling their conditions. They wonder, *Are creating goals and planning a future even options for me?*

For children who face medical conditions, we should always be searching for how we can help them visualize their futures. Even easily treatable injuries can have long-term effects if we don't approach them in a hopeful way and alleviate emotional trauma.

Hope even leaves its mark in the most desperate times. I saw that happen in New

Orleans after Hurricane Katrina. I have never heard more people say, "God bless you," without anyone sneezing, than I did when I volunteered in New Orleans after that devastating storm.

During my time volunteering at a center there, I met Jasmine. She was almost four years old and a bright little girl. We bounced a basketball back and forth as we worked on math problems. We also reviewed the alphabet, and I helped her practice spelling a short list of words. Jasmine needed to know that her world was going to return to normal someday, that this was just a bump in the road. As I always say, "It's going to

> *It's going to be a speed bump in the rearview mirror at some point.*

be a speed bump in the rearview mirror at some point."

I think the person who gave me the best perspective on life in New Orleans was Agnes, an eighty-three-year-old African American woman. As part of my work, I travelled to Agnes's nursing home to make sure all of the patients had their medications and that their blood sugar levels and vitals were stable. A lot of the residents were stranded at this location, and the home had just a few employees to take care of them. Agnes and I were sitting at a table talking while I checked her blood pressure. She told me she had been trapped on the third floor in the middle of the hurricane when the power failed. She was in her wheelchair. With no electricity, she couldn't come down on the elevator.

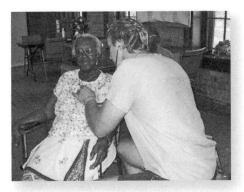

Agnes said, "Honey, I was living through these long
before they started naming them."

"So I sat there and watched the storm through the window the whole night," she said.

"Agnes, that must have been terrifying."

She patted me on the forearm and said, "Honey, I was living through these long before they started naming them."

The people of New Orleans gave me hope, and we tried to do the same for them. Our group of volunteers from Indianapolis consisted of students, firefighters, pastors, police officers, doctors, nurses, moms, dads, and members of a motorcycle gang. Everybody just piled into a bus and headed south. We used seven tractor-trailers to carry loads of necessities for the people we hoped to help. The trucks followed our bus as we drove toward New Orleans.

Most of the trip was uneventful through Kentucky and Tennessee. Once we reached Alabama, we were shocked to see, probably five days after the hurricane, trees still lying across the highways—not just the back roads but the main interstate.

It looked like the flooded skeletal remains of a city with the amount of damage and devastation. Buildings had been ripped apart, flattened, as if by explosions. It was shocking to see a city the size of New Orleans under water. You know it's a real disaster when even the McDonald's is closed. The city had declared martial law, which was, incidentally, why we were able to practice medicine there.

> *You know it's a real disaster when even the McDonald's is closed.*

People often ask, "Why don't you do more of what you practice in other countries with Timmy Global Health in the United States?" We'd be happy to, but legally we can't. Many of the trial lawyers, or "limousine liberals," as I like to call them, want to maintain their ability to sue healthcare providers. To practice in a state, you have to be licensed in that particular state. If martial law has been declared, the state/city can give clearance for doctors and nurses from other states to come into the area to practice medicine. I recently was involved in the passage of House Bill 1145 in the state of Indiana. The bill will give some medical malpractice protection to healthcare providers who volunteer to provide care to the underserved. I am pleased that other states have passed such laws and several more states are considering such legislation. But it saddens me that we now have to create legislation to protect people who are trying to do good.

New Orleans was like a sci-fi movie about the end of the world. It didn't seem like a place where we would be encountering hope, but it was. The worst had already happened, and we were helping by taking care of people in whatever way we could.

One of the people I treated was an older gentleman who had diabetes. I was concerned about his blood sugar getting out of control. He had no electricity in his home, and it was hot and humid. He was sitting out in the middle of his yard, so I did a house call underneath his shade tree. There were flies and bugs swarming around him, but he was appreciative. We sat and talked as I treated his medical needs. Frankly, it's wonderful when I can help other people without the necessity of documenting it all, as we must in conventional healthcare arenas in the United States.

I have seen the best in people after disasters. I experienced people's kindness and generosity after 9/11. I witnessed it after Hurricane Katrina. We have nowhere to turn but to God and each other in those times. That trip confirmed for me, again, the power of the human spirit.

Many of my patients have been through devastating situations. Imagine that you're suddenly quadriplegic. You might not be able to take a breath on your own or bathe yourself anymore. You have lost the ability to use your arms. There doesn't seem to be any reason to have hope in such a situation. Yet, you have to reach the point where you realize it's all about your spirit, your state of mind. It's about living a faithful life and believing something good can come out of the worst circumstances.

Whether you're taking care of an individual patient or working on public health issues, the need for hope is the same. You must encourage a population to rebuild or heal just as you do an individual. Your mere presence in those circumstances can give people hope. They, and you, will never forget what you provided for each other.

SEEKING REFUGE

Arbner was a ten-year-old boy I met while working with Kosovar refugees in Durres, Albania. I had been asked by Muslim Hope to go to Durres with the executive director of their foundation to help set up a clinic that would supply long-term medical care to the refugees. When I entered the refugee camp, a young boy ran up and grabbed my arm. It was Arbner. He was wearing a Kosovo Liberation Army beret. He thought I was there to help fight the Serbs. Through a translator, I explained I was a medical doctor who had come to help with the relief effort.

Arbner insisted on leading me through the camp. He also introduced me to all of his friends and family. As we walked, it was obvious that Arbner had made many friends throughout the camp. He seemed to enjoy being part of the effort to help people from his community. During my stay, I became his friend, too.

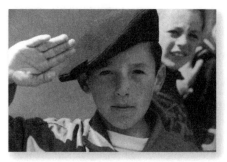

Arbner

Finally, it came time for me to leave the camp. Arbner insisted on having several photos taken with me. When we reached the gate, the guard wouldn't let him exit with me. We hugged before I walked through the gate. Arbner pulled free from the guard and ran to our car. My last memory of him was him standing at the car window, saluting me with tears in his eyes. Tears also flowed from my eyes then and now, as I relate this story.

I tell students, "You can go back to the villages we visited in other countries where they have little to nothing, no electricity or water. As many as ten or twenty years later, they will still remember you. You showed up and gave them hope by being there to share the experience with them."

CHAPTER 12

Be Amazed

We've lost our sense of awe. We seem to think we have the answers to all of life's mysteries. Yet we are only describing what we can observe and measure. When we look at the workings of each organ of the body, each cell within that organ, each molecule within the cell, we don't fully understand how or why they function. We barely scratch the surface of understanding.

I have been asked, "Have you ever seen the miraculous? Have you ever seen something remarkable?" I reply, "Every birth of a child is miraculous." When we see an occurrence repeatedly, we begin to take it for granted. As my friend, a country song-writer, stated in one of his songs, "It's hard to see

Every birth of a child is miraculous.

the picture when you're in the frame." We lose perspective. When working in other countries, without the medications and technology available in the United States, I am more aware of miraculous events.

The human spirit is amazing to me. So are the children I care for, especially considering their limitations caused by disease or disability.

Stephen R. Covey said, "We are not human beings on a spiritual journey. We are spiritual beings on a human journey." I wonder if that awareness is cultural or dependent upon how each of us developed, regardless of where in the world we were born. I sometimes feel we become less aware as we age, rather than more aware.

The Zen teacher Thich Nhat Hanh says we're here to awaken from the illusion of our separateness. I don't believe I ever had that illusion. I've always known how inter-connected we all are. It's astonishing to me when people don't see how connected and similar we are. Even though we are unique in terms of our race, creed, color, abilities, gender, etc., we are all human. In fact, the similarities that unite us as human beings, in spite of all that is unique about each person, allow us to experience amazement in our daily lives. Amazement keeps us young at heart.

EXPERIENCE AMAZEMENT THROUGH THE EYES OF A CHILD

If you hike in a field or go to a stream with a child who has never had an intimate experience with nature, watch his sense of awe. It will help bring back your own sense of awe. You will also find that the more time you spend with children, the more you will reconnect with your true, pure soul.

Children need to have lofty goals that they think are near impossible to attain. When we help them reach those goals, it makes a huge difference in how they interact with the world. I don't want my kids going to physical therapy, occupational therapy, and speech therapy every day without having some ultimate goal. One thing I have always done in the social history on all my medical charts is ask patients, "What's something you want to do that you can't imagine getting to do? What's your ultimate wish? What's your dream?" They always have a wish.

I met Todd about twenty years ago. At the time, he was a ten-year-old boy who had never had the opportunity to be treated by a doctor in our specialty. As a result, he was very spastic; his muscles and movements tight. During my first meeting with him, his mom and dad went through his history with me. The whole time, Todd shook with laughter. He grew so spastic from his laughter he would have popped out of his wheelchair if it hadn't been for his seatbelt. "Why is he laughing so much?" I asked. The nurse informed me that he couldn't wait to meet Doctor Doom. He had already been told that I was also a professional wrestler.

I said to his mom, "Why don't you unbuckle him, and I'll suplex him onto the mat here." I didn't have exam tables in my rooms. I had big mats where I crawled around and stretched out the kids to measure their ranges of motion and the tightness of their muscles from muscle diseases and brain or spinal cord injuries. She unbuckled him, and I pulled him up from the wheelchair. He went straight into extension: up on his toes because of the spasticity. Knowing I wouldn't hurt him, I decided to do a wrestling move called a vertical suplex on him. I grabbed him in a reverse headlock and flipped him in the air over my right shoulder and onto the mat. I sat back up and looked at his mom and dad, who stared at me as if to say, "What the hell was that?" Tough Todd, on the other hand, lay there laughing so hard he couldn't breathe. I told him he was starting to look like a Smurf and needed to take a breath.

That was the beginning. Three weeks later, we had our first-ever professional wrestling show where the kids were the stars. I was helped by my rugby buddy, Brian Burhenn, who is also known as "Cargo." Cargo is six feet, seven inches tall, and he weighed 340 pounds at the time. (Brian has become the children's favorite amusement ride.) The whole purpose of the wrestling show was to convince the children that the focus was no longer on their disabilities but on their abilities—

their abilities to entertain through their creativity and the use of whatever parts of their bodies worked.

I wanted those kids to have bragging rights when they went back to school after the weekend. When their friends discussed what they had done, they might say, "Oh, I watched the football game." Or "I watched cartoons." Or "I played Xbox with my friends." But these children could say, "I was a pro wrestler Saturday." There aren't too many kids who get to boast about that.

LIFE ITSELF IS A DEATH-DEFYING ACT

I've always viewed these opportunities as opening the door for kids. How do I get them through the door? The minute I flipped Todd over my head onto the mat, I thought, *We need to do this.* We needed to show the parents, "Yes, these kids are fragile but not that breakable." Thus was born the event that would eventually become the Timmy Takedown.

Some people think we push the limits too much. I started giving a presentation called "Life Itself Is a Death-Defying Act." I tried to explain that if we're going to be here, we ought to live passionately. These kids deserve to be in the spotlight, and that's what we do for them. We create all types of events and use our connections within the community and sports world to make their dreams become reality.

We had twenty-five kids the first time we organized a wrestling show. There were crash pads and lots of space in the gym where we were holding the event. The kids came in the gym where they often did their physical therapy. It wasn't fancy. We tumbled around and explained to them how to do some pro wrestling moves. We tossed them, lifted them up, and dropped them. We did some suplexes and power slams, but as we came through the movements, we gently laid the children to the mats.

Before that first show, a little boy wearing a flannel shirt and blue jeans looked up at Cargo. The boy's mouth fell open, and his eyes gawked. He slowly scanned Brian, from his legs all the way up to his head, which to the boy must have seemed to be up to the ceiling. Brian gathered the little boy's flannel shirt with his massive right hand and lifted that two-year-old up until he was level with Brian's head —six feet, seven inches.

"Don't think I'm going to take it easy on you because you're a kid," Brian said.

He then sat the boy back down and kept on walking.

If the boy was frightened, he didn't show it. In fact, I have noticed that despite all the things we say and do, these kids are never intimidated. I am concerned one of them may break into tears. A few have gotten scared, but they all overcome it, especially when they enter the ring where they see and hear all the people cheering for them. The bigger the show, the more exciting it becomes. Their families love it, and the community loves it. Recently we brought in professional wrestlers from World Wrestling Entertainment (WWE), which prompted more interest in the program. We even had a local radio celebrity, Ray Steele, volunteer to help us. His daughter's ring moniker is the Mad Scientist.

The kids love getting into the wrestling ring. I went to one elementary school to put on a wrestling show that would feature Susie, a little girl who had Down syndrome. I was told that she didn't like loud noises and that the place "must be totally quiet when she comes in." I agreed to try to keep everyone quiet. There were 450 or more students and faculty in this gym, and they sat there so quietly you could hear Susie's tentative footsteps.

Susie entered the gym and looked around. She was surprised to see so many people. She climbed into the ring. I encouraged everyone to stay quiet, and then I whispered to her. We did the walking and talking that we do in professional wrestling. I told her what to do. She grabbed and twisted my arm. I did a flip and landed on my back. The audience couldn't restrain their elation. The place erupted. They cheered and yelled her name. Suddenly, this little girl who didn't like loud noises marched around, arms joyfully extended, and celebrated the feeling that everybody was shouting her name. Loud noises are okay with her now, as long as people are chanting "Susie!"

The event belongs to the children. They must come up with their own wrestling personas, ring names, and costumes. And they all have to have a finishing move, a move that brings the crowd to their feet cheering as they win their matches and earn their championship belts. The whole show becomes dependent on the development of each character that each child creates. Are we going to carry them in on a throne? What sort of confetti do they need? Parents love it because they help design the costumes. Student volunteers for Timmy Global Health make signs, toss confetti, and blow horns and do creative lighting. It's a big show these days.

When I travel to Mexico each year for clinics, I bring back a bag full of professional wrestling masks to give to the kids. I encourage them even while they're in the hospital. "Hey, we've got this big show coming up. You need to be a part of it." It serves as a goal beyond the immediate challenge they're facing. In rehabilitation, we outline short-term goals leading to long-term goals. We need to have a vision for what we ultimately try to achieve in any situation. What does the best possible outcome look like? It usually exceeds what most people could imagine.

Once the day of the event arrives, everything needs to be built around it. We rent a place that is accessible for people with any disabilities. All the levels of the space are wheelchair accessible, so the kids and fans can get around easily. The show begins before we're even in the gymnasium, which is how it should be. This is the fun part for me. We're all dressed and ready. We talk to the kids, and the excitement builds. Some are nervous because they've never performed in front of a crowd.

Brian and I usually kneel down with the kids around us and say, "Now remember, this is like the amusement park. If you get in the roller coaster, you have to keep your arms and legs inside. If we tuck your arms and legs in, keep your head down. We're going to flip or toss you, so stay safe."

To some of the kids who have little to no movement, we say, "You just turn our fingers. We'll jump, go airborne, and land splat, and then you just pin us." Cargo, Mighty Joe, or I will pick the child up and sit him across the other wrestler's chest for the pin.

"Remember we're not really going to kick and hit," I tell them. "We're just tumbling. We're doing gymnastics here. This is all that therapy you've been doing. This is where it's really going to pay off. We're going to do flips, rolls, and tosses. You might win this match!"

Then I ask, "Any questions?" Most times, they don't have any questions. But their parents often have reminders—naturally— for me. One time, three mothers leaned into the huddle.

"Chuck, don't forget Sydney just had that hip redone three weeks ago," one of them said. "Don't dislocate her hip."

Another mother advised, "Bobby had that G-tube replaced. Make sure you don't pull it out while you're wrestling."

"Yeah, Doctor Doom," a third mother chimed in, "Jill had that urology procedure. They just put her catheter in again. Make sure you don't pull that out."

I love the fact that with those few precautions, none of the mothers were saying don't do this or this isn't a good idea. It deeply moves me when a parent hands a child, unable to move, through the ropes to participate in our show. I always tell parents we'll take the greatest care of their children.

Another great part of the Timmy Takedown experience is that it gives these children the opportunity to give back. We have sponsorships and charge a small amount for people to attend the event. Because these children have disabilities, they receive disability benefits. They are often Medicaid patients, so they rely on tax dollars and others to help take care of them. This is their time to return that blessing. They help raise money to take care of children in US and other countries who are in the same situation. Here is the opportunity for the Timmy Takedown heroes to make a difference in the world.

This is typically not a big fundraiser. We may make $5,000 or $6,000. One year, we had a guy come to the show who thought it was great. He walked from the stands and handed our executive director a check for $5,000. Suddenly, it *was* a big fundraiser. It's a heartwarming, positive family experience that permeates well beyond what happens that day. I try to make sure these kids are aware of how they've affected the world.

Young men and women who previously participated in the wrestling show return to help the younger kids. They show the new wrestlers they can succeed and help them highlight their abilities. Some work as referees. Others help coach the young wrestlers. Some have been tag team partners with us, wrestling the kids. They help create the opportunity for the children to be successful at showcasing their abilities.

When the event is over, people often tell us, "I laughed. I cried. I couldn't believe it. It was the greatest thing I've ever seen." One man told me, "I've been a fan of pro wrestling for thirty years... This was the greatest wrestling show I've seen!"

That's the reaction we hope to get. We *want* them to have a sense of amazement. We *want* them to leave the show saying,

"Wow, these kids are remarkable. Look what they can do."

I wish we did Timmy Takedown every day. There are enough kids that we could do it more often. We have to change our philosophies about how we treat patients. We have to think like a child to make therapies more fun and creative. I would love to have a full-time gym with a professional wrestling ring in it. In that setting, the kids wouldn't just be going to physical therapy and occupational therapy; they'd be going to the gym. "I have to go work out today because I'm a pro wrestler."

That would be amazing.

And here's one more amazing part of all the years we've put on Timmy Takedown: Doctor Doom and Cargo have lost more than six hundred matches in a row. But who's counting?

CHAPTER 13

Be an Instrument of Peace

I once met a young man from Russia while I was volunteering at a children's camp. During our conversation, he was surprised to hear that I had been to his country. He was even more stunned when he learned that I had paid to travel there to help people. I have noticed that people who live or have lived under a communist government can be suspicious of my motives. So I took it in stride when he asked me about my motivation for my assistance in his homeland.

"Well, my faith dictates I care for others," I told him. "That is why I became a doctor, to take care of the children."

I have never viewed my choice to become a doctor as an opportunity to become wealthy off the misery of others. And when I am asked to explain the ultimate goal of Timmy Global Health, I like to hold my finger to my head, as if I have to contemplate the answer. Finally, I say, "How about world peace?"

I firmly believe that the work we do at Timmy Global Health is the path to peace. If I could, I would introduce to the world all the children in my care. I'm convinced that children with challenges and disabilities make us more compassionate and more humane. If people could spend time with these children and care for them, I have no doubt there would be more peace and less prejudice in the world.

I believe that, even while knowing there is great hatred in the world. An elderly Serbian woman once told our team, "You Americans do not understand why we hate each other. We've hated each other not for decades or centuries, we have hated each other for millennia."

I also will never forget the comment I heard when I worked with the Kosovar refugees at a children's hospital in Albania. One day, the Albanian medical director said to me, "Good news, Dr. Chuck. Four babies were born last night: one girl and three soldiers."

Yet I have also encountered hope.

During the fall of 1992, in the early part of my career, I had the opportunity to go on my first trip to help with a new healthcare in the former Soviet Union. I went to Moscow, St. Petersburg, and Tallinn, Estonia. While I was there, I spent time in the Institute of Traumatology, the large trauma center in Moscow. I cared for several children who had been in a train accident when they traveled between the Ural Mountains and Moscow. One train collided with another train, causing a gas pipeline near the train tracks to explode and ignite an inferno. Many children died. The survivors were the ones I worked with in the hospital. They sure didn't look like enemies of the state.

During that time, I met some young, compassionate Russian doctors who were genuinely committed to the people of their country. They had not yet seen a free market. How would they know what a healthcare system looks like within a free market? I set up a program to bring these doctors to the United States to gather support for their work. I said, "It is important that you speak adequate English, can tell your story, and appeal to people who can support you." I had one of the doctors bring Russian artwork to the United States each time he visited. We encouraged people in the American communities to come to Russian art shows and contribute financial support to these doctors to get the resources they needed to help patients in their country.

THE POLITICS OF PEACE

Politicians have their own agendas— agendas that often interfere with the work of healthcare professionals and caregivers. It's my belief that if we could get politicians out of the way, we could interact with people from other countries much more productively. We would discover that we really have a lot in common with people we have been told are our enemies. That is what happened during my visit to the former Soviet Union. I developed many friendships. Interacting face to face with the citizens of other nations reveals how similar we are in our dreams, desires, and needs. And nothing bonds us more than our children.

To show up in any location and heal children diffuses a lot of suffering and anger. It can even diffuse hatred. I've been in places—Macedonia, for example—where hatred of one population was palpable and extremely uncomfortable for me. But I know that even the most hard-hearted people can be softened by children. If there is generational hatred between two populations, it is difficult to intervene at the level of the adults to make a difference. Yet if you heal their children, that softens the hearts of the parents and grandparents. You also inspire a new, more peaceful worldview among the younger generation you're helping to heal.

Years ago, some students asked me, "What would you do if you were elected president?"

I said, "That's easy. The first thing I would do is I'd reinstitute the draft."

It was fun to just sit and watch their puzzled reactions for a moment.

"What I have in mind," I continued, "is that as Americans finish high school—whether they drop out or graduate—we send them off to countries to heal, rather than to kill, others."

If we did that, there would be an incredible amount of healing going on between many countries. The perceptions some countries' residents have of the United States would change, and the perceptions within the United States of what other peoples are like would also change. Another advantage is that our young people would see how much they have, simply by being born in this country.

I once shared this philosophy during a talk I gave at a church. After my talk, a distinguished, older gentleman came up to me as the crowd cleared. In a private moment, he said, "Dr. Chuck, I listened to what you had to say today. I was in the US military for a long time, and I'm very proud of what I did for our country. But I believe what you said today made the most sense about our having world peace someday, and I'd like you to have this." He gave me his Special Forces coin, a gift I treasure to this day. It's a reminder of all the good people I've met who also hope for peace.

CHAPTER 14

Be an Inspiration

One of the projects of Timmy Global Health that has made a huge impact is the Bebor Primary School in Nigeria. The school cost $12,000 to build, and 260 students attend it. They do not have a gymnasium or an indoor pool, but they're getting an education. A full year's tuition and a school uniform costs

$51. I'm happy to report we have as many girls on scholarships as boys. That's important in a traditionally patriarchal, polygamous culture. The school uniforms are made by their mothers. Both the boys and the girls wear pink.

> *A full year's tuition and a school uniform costs $51.*

That kind of educational undertaking is how we'll solve problems of poverty and build a better world. These are our young students, the people we're mentoring. Keep that in mind. They're going to be taking over for us someday. My favorite St. Francis quote is: "Preach the Gospel at all times, and when necessary use words." It's important for all of us to remember that children get their greatest instruction from watching adults. We can say what we like, but they're watching to see how we actually act.

When I studied pediatrics as a medical student, a mural in one of the clinics was emblazoned with the words, "Children learn what they live." I remember seeing that adage and thinking, *They also live what they learn.* Why am I so committed to this kind of work, and why do I give so much? That's how my parents lived. That's what I learned from watching them. It isn't easy taking on such responsibility. As Mother Teresa used to say, "I am a little pencil in God's hands."

My dad tended to be obsessive-compulsive. He wanted the house to be orderly— everything in its place. That didn't happen with a bunch of kids in the house. Thankfully, he lived long enough for us to talk about it. I matured enough to tell him how impressed I was by what he was willing to sacrifice, including his desire for orderliness, to provide for that many kids who came into our home.

I was also impressed with my mom, who gave well beyond the point at which most people are comfortable. She could give even

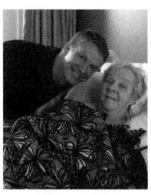

when it became painful. She cared for any child in need, whether that child was one of her biological children, one in our community, or one of the

My Maternal Mentor

foster children. We might have three foster babies in the home at any given time. That kind of sacrifice takes great commitment.

ART OR SCIENCE

In retrospect, I have to say I'm a hybrid of my parents. My ability with numbers and my obsessive-compulsive traits have helped make me a good doctor. It's important for me to use my scientific mind for a good cause, not to gain title or money. Those aren't things that appeal to me or motivate me. But I have come to understand that money is an important resource. It is not the most important resource in our work, but it is typically the most limiting.

When I was a resident doctor, the chairman of our department challenged us at a conference. He asked, "Is medicine an art or a science?" I quickly replied, "That's easy. Medicine is the art of the application of our science." But I knew he wasn't going to let us choose both. It had to be one or the other. He and everyone else in the room chose science. I chose art.

I sat in the conference room thinking about the placebo effect and the power of being present. You can make a huge difference by supporting people, being there, touching them, and telling them that you believe in them. That's an art form. We live in the world of Western medicine where we have all these medicines and procedures, but I still stand by my belief that some of the most powerful medicine cannot be quantified.

I felt vindicated when a friend shared an experience he had in Africa. "You know, Chuck," he said, "I thought I had such a great day at the

> *Medicine is the art of the application of our science.*

252

clinic. I spent the whole day working. I bet I saw 100 to 120 patients. As they came through, I scribbled their diagnoses and what medicines I was dispensing as I handed them their medicine. At the end of the day, I walked outside the building, and all the medicine was lying in a big pile on the ground outside the door."

He shared what went wrong, starting with the fact that he was right-handed. As he wrote down the diagnoses and the names of the medicines he distributed—so he could be better prepared on the next trip— he handed people their medicines with his left hand. In a culture in which there are no hygienic toileting areas or toilet paper, the left hand is considered dirty. People use their left hands to clean themselves by splashing water around their bottoms after going to the bathroom. Anything given with the left hand to another person is considered worthless and dirty. There's your science lying on the ground outside the clinic because the art of healing in that culture was lacking.

SIMPLE MOMENTS INSPIRE US, TOO

Children are watching. They're seeing how we do what we do, including how we practice the art of medicine. Are we supportive? Are we giving enough of ourselves?

Amanda was a little girl with cerebral palsy. It affected her legs, making them very tight and weak. At first, she could only crawl to move around, but after repeated sessions of therapy, she was using a rolling walker. The next step was even harder—trying to walk with the use of forearm crutches. She struggled to get used to them. One day in clinic, when she was five, I asked her if she could show me what she could do with her crutches. With her angelic, little face, she looked up at me, looked at her parents, and said, "Okay." She then spit on her hands, rubbed them together, and proceeded to get up and walk across the room with her new pink crutches.

It's those small moments that can make a difference. When I'm at the local children's hospital here in the United States or in a remote location somewhere in the world, I always take the stethoscope out of my ears and put it in the ears of the children I'm examining. I want them to listen to my heart, to their hearts, to their parents' and siblings' hearts. I want them to see that although we may not look the same, we may be different colors, we may speak different languages and have different creeds, what ticks within us—how we function, our desires, needs, and love for each other—is universal. We are 99.99999 percent the same.

That brief moment of taking the stethoscope out of my ears and putting it into the ears of a child might also inspire a future healer. That child might remember that moment and become a nurse, doctor, public health provider, or community health worker for her village. Small moments can be significant enough to make kids entertain the possibility of giving of themselves to heal another.

I saw that happen in a special way when I once visited a church in Indianapolis to invite people to be a part of this work. Within two days of speaking there, I received an envelope in the mail. I opened

it and found a letter wrapped around fif-
ty-nine dollars cash, stuffed in the envelope.
The letter was obviously written by a child's
hand. When I read it, I was moved and
amazed.

The child wrote,
"Dear Dr. Chuck,
You probably don't
remember me. I was
at a talk you made at
St. Luke Catholic. I

*We are
99.99999
percent the
same.*

was very touched by your talk. However,
I'm not old enough to go around the world
helping people with you. However, I hope
what I'm enclosing can help you. Also, I'm
not including my name. If you would, just
call me Z. Hope this helps.

Sincerely, Z.

P.S.: I haven't included any coins. They
make too much noise."

Z is exactly what we are looking for at Timmy Global Health, a child with a big heart—compassionate but practical and logical about how we can accomplish our mission of helping others. At that time, Z did not feel he or she was ready to go and do this global work, but Z emptied the piggy bank and sent me the funds, so we could do our work as his or her ambassador.

The good news is, despite the donor remaining anonymous, the envelope had a last name and return address on it. That $59 in cash was sacred. I couldn't even bring myself to take the money out of the envelope and deposit it at the bank. I carried it to state and national conferences to tell people the story, and I read the letter to them until it almost fell apart. I kept it in the envelope. I said, "You need to handle this. It's sacred. Pass it around."

Every time that envelope circulated through any auditorium where I spoke, it came back with hundreds, if not thousands, of dollars. People were moved by what Z had done. For years, I wrote to Z at the return address on the envelope. "Dear Z," I would write, "just so you know, here's how you've changed the world. You've touched many people. I want you to know about this."

About seven years after I received Z's letter, I participated in a charity walkathon in Indianapolis. During the walk, I introduced myself to a woman. She said, "I know. You're Dr. Chuck. You came and spoke at our church."

"What church is that?" I asked.

"St. Luke Catholic Church," she answered. When she shared her last name, it was the same as Z's. So I asked her if she lived on the street that Z had included on the envelope's return address.

"How would you know that?" she asked.

"Well, I feel I'm betraying somebody," I said. "But I think a mother would want to know this."

I told her about the letter and money from Z, who was her daughter. She was surprised and proud of what her daughter had done.

Z's gift is an example of how you need to "find your own Calcutta," as Mother Teresa used to say. You can change the world right in your community. You can also change the world at large by supporting someone who goes out as your ambassador. I look forward to the day when Z joins us in our work in the field.

IN THE PRESENCE
OF GREATNESS

I am blessed to have incredible, synergistic relationships with my patients. I had a patient, Tyler, who has cerebral palsy. One day, I walked outside with his mother after we had finished a clinic visit. She said, "Are you aware of the energy in that room when you're with my son?" I said, "Yes, I am. That's why I do what I do."

It's a powerful experience to be the caregiver of my spiritual leaders. To me, it's been worth giving up other opportunities in life. Great, heroic acts happen all the time in the hospitals and clinics where I see kids. To be in the presence of greatness is worth sacrificing many things. I've witnessed children take their first steps after a brain injury. I've been there when a child came out of a coma, regained the ability to speak, and was able to say to his mother, "I love you." I've had the opportunity to talk with children who have died, been resuscitated, and came back to tell me there was nothing to fear. My little gurus often break my heart and then repair it in one encounter.

> *My little gurus often break my heart and then repair it in one encounter.*

BIG INSPIRATIONS COME IN SMALL PACKAGES

As a doctor, I've experienced life-saving events. Simple moments can also be deeply moving. It's inspiring to see what other people are willing to forgo for the sake of someone in need, such as what a mother will do for her child. I remember one little boy in Ecuador. Sebastian was one year old, and he had a life-threatening illness. We needed to find out what surgeries and medications were needed to save his life. I tried to encourage his mother. "We will do whatever is necessary," I said. She began to cry. I cried, too. I find it terribly difficult to witness a mother cry for her child. These children belong to all of us.

A colleague had an experience in Haiti as he was delivering food to a family.

The father thanked my friend, took the food, and gave it all to his children. As he watched them eat, the father said, "They're still growing. They need to eat every day. I only need to eat every other day."

I often get to experience such inspirational moments in my work. I've also seen heroic acts performed by people who have traveled with me. While we tried to save the life of an infant in Haiti, one of our doctors was exposed to HIV through a needle stick. We contacted an infectious disease doctor by satellite phone. He directed us to begin the antiviral treatment. As a team, we had to remain focused on taking care of the Haitian people while also addressing our own needs. The safety of the team is paramount, or no one gets treated.

Our medical team saw a four-year old child in Ecuador who had shingles. He was wearing a tight-fitting, dirty shirt. As we peeled off his shirt, it was clear that the lesions were very painful. We completed our exam and outlined the treatment plan for his mother. As we were preparing him to leave, one of the students could not bear the thought of the pain caused by replacing his shirt. The young man pulled off his T-shirt and placed it over the child's head, covering his trunk. The boy looked like an angelic figure, now that he had donned a white robe.

There's also the reality that some of the treatments we've had to perform to heal kids haven't been easy. Some procedures have even been painful for the child, but knowing that is even a greater motivator to ensure we accomplish what we set out to do. We have to step across that threshold, always believing the child will be healed.

THE FUTURE OF INSPIRATION

I'm very impressed by the younger gen-
erations. I lecture to young people from
kindergarten through medical school. I'm
inspired by them. I try to nurture their
talents, potential, and compassion. And
I think they get it. They understand they
could pursue money, power, and titles, but
it's an empty pursuit. Real spiritual growth
will come from accepting their roles in
healing the world and helping other people.

I want these young people to be better
than me. I had a friend Sister Bernadette.
She had been a cloistered nun for more
than eighty-four years. My mother went
to her for prayerful support when I was
going to Albania to work with the Kosovar
refugees. Sister Bernadette said, "Poor Dr.

Chuck. His heart is bigger than his brain." I'm happy to proclaim that the healers of this next generation have both big hearts and big brains. Because of this combination, the world is going to be healthier in the future.

Conclusion

Be Persistent

We live in a culture filled with cynicism and negativity. It's important to try to stay above those reactions and attitudes. When Mother Teresa talked about improving the world and helping individuals, she told people to find their own Calcutta. She encouraged people to work with those closest to them. We have family members and friends in our own homes and communities who need assistance. People are not always called to do this work on a global scale. In the United States, we tend to talk about "global" health as though it does not include our country. Yes, the United States is part of the globe.

Mother Teresa pointed out that the greatest affliction is people not feeling wanted. She noticed that in extended care facilities in the US, people sat and watched the door, hoping for someone to visit them. I realized at a young age that we all have an inherent need to be needed. That's how we stay connected to one another. I do not understand how one may have the desire for isolation. We are all connected in our hearts, though we need to be reminded of that bond on occasion. There is a piece of eternity, of God, within each of us that longs for that connection.

I have a special connection of the heart with the children I care for, whether they're here in the United States or somewhere around the world. I've learned it's important to communicate with them to find out what they need to improve their health and assure their development. I feel more alive when I'm serving them and meeting their needs. It energizes me even more to watch children who have benefited from our support take on nurturing roles. They often become caregivers of other children in need. When they have endured suffering, they learn to be empathetic and thus compassionate. They can say, "I know where you are, I've been there, and I will help you through this because others were there for me."

Patients tell me I'm not just their doctor but also their friend. I try to help them through their challenges and difficulties, to offer them some kind of healing. Still, I have to admit that trying to provide this healing can sometimes chip away at my heart, especially when kids don't make it. These hardships have taken their toll on me. They've made me contemplate how much personal cost has been involved in my choices and how pursuing this kind of work has affected my personal relationships. I sometimes wonder if I can continue on this path or if it's time to step down.

At the same time, when I'm in the field taking risks and going to dangerous places with limited resources, life speeds up for me. I've always had this dream of throwing some medicine and cash into a bag and wandering the planet to take care of children. I've done that in a way, but I have also considered what it would be like to continue rambling for a long time and not necessarily return to a home base. It would be an interesting journey, stripping down to some of the basics you think you need and leaving home to deliver medicine and healing—just to see what good comes of it. I have no doubt I would encounter many people in need. It's always a wonderful experience to show up with the necessary resources to save a child and offer hope to a family.

That goal has always been the priority for Timmy Global Health. Now, I would like to see our efforts grow even more. In the next few years, I hope we can double the number of our international partners and also the number of chapters we have in high schools and colleges. I'm hoping to travel more to spread our philosophy and spend more time with students in the United States and abroad. I encourage them to become mentors, and I enjoy handing the reins to them.

My other hope is that the healthcare system in the United States can be changed. As I travel around, lecturing on the mission of healthcare, or stressing the importance of making a difference, I talk to healthcare professionals. I thank them for their commitments. I encourage them to work with me to move toward a healthcare system that focuses more on delivery of care than documentation of care. I always get a positive response. Yet, unfortunately, our industry continues to look more like a business than a mission. Long ago, Plato recognized the difference between a healing mission and business. He penned *The Republic* in 380 B.C. In the dialogue, he inquired, "But tell me, this physician of whom you were just speaking, is he a moneymaker, an earner of fees, or a healer of the sick?" My hope is to encourage healthcare systems at every level to become refocused on the patients who have been entrusted to our care.

I remember driving around Indianapolis and seeing billboards advertising "patient-focused care." I thought, *What else would you focus on?* The fact that we even have to see a marketing tagline like that is deeply discouraging. Healthcare has evolved so far in the wrong direction in our country that we have to remind our providers that their focus should be on the patients. Instead, we are distracted by our computers, data, reimbursement, prior authorizations, liability, protocols, and policies.

We need to get back to that cornerstone of why we became doctors, nurses, therapists, and pharmacists. All the other concerns would fall into place. Most importantly, we would deliver better care and do a better job of healing patients.

It's easy to believe that when we encounter people in need, we'll just give medicine or perform surgical procedures necessary to improve their lives. My students quickly learn that healing is a mutual experience. Henri Nouwen does a wonderful job of addressing this point in his book, *The Wounded Healer*. What we bring into the arena—our life experiences, our spiritual journeys, our loves and losses, and our heart-aches—makes us better healers. Too often, we attempt to keep our patients at arm's length. Extending our arms, embracing our patients, and bringing them closer leads to a healing experience for both of us.

That approach guided the life and the caring mission of Mother Teresa. The ripple effect of that approach continues to spread in the lives of the people who are carrying Mother Teresa medallions, the ones that have a thread from her sari. And fortunately, it doesn't end there. There is a common thread that binds everyone who offers hope and healing to another person.

I have aspired to be a source of hope and healing for the children who have been in my care, just as their magnificent spirits have been a source of hope and healing for me. At this point, their stories have been woven into my story, the story now in front of you.

Thank you for opening your heart to my spiritual heroes…

Thank you for allowing your heart to be broken…

Thank you for wrapping your heart around your mission.